Not since the 1940s has there been such uncertainty within and about
Europe. Who can tell what the map will look like by the turn of the century?
What will be the pattern of economic performance? Whose vision of the best
way to run a society will prevail? *New Perspectives on the Welfare State in
Europe* focuses on this last facet of uncertainty. It examines welfare statism
and our present understanding of it, compares the welfare state in Europe
with those elsewhere in the world, and investigates particular trends and
prospects within and across Europe.

The contributors, all leading authorities in the field, explore a variety of
themes. They cover a wide range of topics, including the prospects for the
British welfare state in Europe and the prospects for an EC welfare state; the
trials of the 'model' Swedish welfare state and the tribulations of former
communist regimes in Eastern Europe; the challenge of Confucianism from
Asia Pacific.

By taking stock of the current situation and weighing future possibilities,
New Perspectives on the Welfare State in Europe provides a timely account
which will be essential reading for students, researchers, lecturers and policy
makers in social policy, politics, and sociology.

Catherine Jones is Reader in Comparative Social Policy at the University
of Birmingham. Among her publications is *Patterns of Social Policy: an
Introduction to Comparative Analysis,* published by Routledge.

New perspectives on the welfare state in Europe

Edited by Catherine Jones

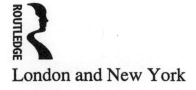

London and New York

First published in 1993
by Routledge
11 New Fetter Lane, London EC4P 4EE
Simultaneously published in the USA and Canada
by Routledge
29 West 35th Street, New York, NY 10001
Reprinted 1996

Typeset in Times by
NWL Editorial Services, Langport, Somerset
Printed and bound in Great Britain by
T. J. Press (Padstow) Ltd, Padstow, Cornwall

British Library Cataloguing in Publication Data
A catalogue record for this book is available from the British Library

Library of Congress Cataloguing in Publication Data
A catalogue record for this book is available from the Library of Congress

ISBN 0–415–07041–4 (hbk)
ISBN 0–415–07042–2 (pbk)

Contents

Illustrations

Contributors

Jonathan Bradshaw: Professor, Department of Social Policy and Social Work, University of York.

Bob Deacon: Reader in Social Policy, Leeds Metropolitan University.

Nicholas Deakin: Professor, Department of Social Policy and Social Work, University of Birmingham.

John Doling: Reader in Housing and Head of Department of Social Policy and Social Work, University of Birmingham.

Arthur Gould: Senior Lecturer, Department of Social Sciences, Loughborough University.

Catherine Jones: Reader in Comparative Social Policy, Department of Social Policy and Social Work, University of Birmingham.

Rudolf Klein: Professor, Centre for the Analysis of Social Policy, University of Bath.

Stephan Leibfried: Professor, German National Science Foundation, University of Bremen.

Ramesh Mishra: Professor, Atkinson College, York University, Ontario.

Jaqi Nixon: Head, Department of Health and Social Studies, Bradford and Ilkley Community College.

Richard Rose: Professor, Centre for the Study of Public Policy, University of Strathclyde.

Valerie Williamson: Principal Lecturer, Department of Community Studies, University of Brighton.

Editorial introduction

Catherine Jones

Not since the 1940s has there been such comprehensive scope for uncertainty within and about Europe. Who knows what the map will look like by the turn of the century; what political structures and alignments will operate; what will be the pattern of economic performance; whose visions of the best way to run a society will prevail? It is with this last facet of uncertainty, exemplified in terms from the most general to the most particular, that the present volume is concerned.

Hence this is a book about welfare statism and our present understanding of it; about welfare state Europe in comparison with elsewhere; about particular welfare state trends and prospects *within and across* Europe; about Britain-in-Europe on the eve of what some see (or intend to see realized) as the European Community's 'social coming of age'.

The idea for the collection originated from the Institute of Contemporary British History. As ideas go in this context, it was distinctly and deliberately open-ended. 'Trends in comparative social policy' was the theme suggested for a conference to be held in Britain, with a view to the eventual publication of a book. There were no limits placed on the interpretation of the theme. As conference convenor I was initially inclined – given the sponsorship and the location of the conference – to start with topical 'British issues' looked at in comparative perspective and from thence to work outwards and upwards, as it were, to issues of Europe and beyond. A second associated objective was to arrive at a collection illustrative of the state of the art of comparative social policy rather than to commission additional pieces of research.

In retrospect, this might well have been a recipe for British parochialism writ large with the aid of 'comparative back-up'. However, two points emerged from the convening of the conference[1] to give a different thrust and direction to the enterprise.

First, my assumption that issues of moment in Britain must necessarily and invariably have been researched in some comparative perspective turned out to be over optimistic. The 1980s into the 1990s may have seemed momentous, even watershed years for the welfare state in Britain, but most of the great debates seem to have taken place in, as it were, comparative isolation. Naturally there was selective reference to foreign example whenever and wherever this seemed to support a particular case – and vice versa. But international ammunition-gathering – or even 'lesson-swapping between friends' as in the case of Thatcher's Britain and Reagan's America – was never the same thing as comparative analysis.

This is a point well made and substantiated by each of the contributors on 'British issues' present in this collection. In every case, albeit to varying extent, the situation they report and reflect is one not merely of research still waiting to be done but of critical questions still waiting to be asked and conceptual frameworks still waiting to be developed. It takes more than a good messenger to disguise (or indeed seek to disguise) this sort of message. It lurks in the background as the subtext in every case, notwithstanding the quality of personal observation, suggestion and prognosis put forward (see below).

The same point is made yet more forcefully, by implication, where there are no messengers to report. Pressure of commitments and other priorities can of course preclude participation by any one individual in a particular project. However, the failure to recruit *at all* on such matters of local moment as (for example) 'parental choice' in education, 'internal markets' in health care or indeed 'consumerism' generally with regard to the public sector, suggests either that the editor/convenor did not look hard enough or that there was not 'enough' to be found – or both. Either way there is a limit to search time and ingenuity – and patience, in the face of too many specialists seemingly put out at the very suggestion that they might or ought to know (or know of someone who knows) anything about their specialism with reference to anywhere outside Britain.

As matters turned out, however, the failure was not critical and might even, in retrospect, be looked on as a blessing in disguise. For the second and *positive* development affecting the thrust of this collection was that, by the time of the conference (May 1991), there were other far more important matters to think about. 'Issues of Europe' were multiplying in urgency and complexity as fast as Thatcherism was turning into yesterday's news even for Britain.

So, instead of a conference about 'Britain, Europe and the World', the end result was a conference that was rather about *Europe* with selective, illustrative *micro* reference to Britain and *macro* reference to elsewhere (North America and the Far East in particular). After which, and reinforced by additional contributions from Professors Mishra and Leibfried[2] respectively, there has emerged this book.

Manifestly this is a collection illustrative of the state of the art of comparative social policy, which, as I have said, was the secondary objective. From literary review to single-issue comparative social politics; from lesson-swapping to futures forecasting; from the comparison of policies and performances on particular fronts to the construction and modification of typologies intended to accommodate (if not account for) every particular: there is something for everyone here.

But wherein lies the unifying theme? There is a sense in which, in this field at any rate, more 'representative' has still to mean less 'homogeneous' in terms of subject matter, less 'consistent' in terms of approach, less 'coherent' in the sense of propounding and sustaining a particular point of view. So in none of these senses is this to be accounted a unified collection. It is rather a series of arguments about comparative social policy, about perspectives on British social policy and above all about social policy trends and prospects in Europe.

There has been no attempt to recruit or select contributors and/or contributions according to points of view. On the contrary – as will become abundantly clear – this is a collection which rather prides itself on *not* having taken a presumptive stance. How else would it be possible to include within the pages of one volume explanatory perspectives so divergent as those (for instance) of Rudolf Klein and Bob Deacon, or priorities so chillingly at odds with one another (in the eyes of this British editor) as those of Stephan Leibfried and Richard Rose?

It is the editor, naturally, who is responsible for the final ordering and grouping of papers. Rudolf Klein and Ramesh Mishra thus open proceedings by commenting each in their inimitable way – though with considerable common ground evident between them – on the past and present quality of our understanding of the modern welfare state and its prospects. There then follows a quartet of papers targeted on specific policy sectors, issues and problems as viewed from a *British*-comparative perspective: Jonathan Bradshaw on the state of our – so far strikingly limited – understanding of social security performance in the context of Europe; John Doling on the promotion of home ownership as a policy priority which (amongst other things) seems to be shifting Britain further *away* from Europe; Nicholas Deakin on the urban planners' instinct, so far, to look to America rather than to Europe for fresh ideas (a cautionary tale); Jaqi Nixon and Valerie Williamson on the significance of policies designed to lure women back to work, considered against the background of measures taken (and not taken) to safeguard the interests of working women in general and working mothers in particular. There then follows the debate in and about Europe *per se*: Stephan Leibfried analyses patterns of state and social policy development as a prelude to estimating the prospects for his own preferred option – a (more German than 'Anglo Saxon') European welfare state-to-be; Arthur Gould reports tellingly on the present troubles of the Swedish welfare state; Bob Deacon supplies timely analysis of past developments and future prospects in countries of Eastern Europe; I offer a 'European perspective' on the rival qualities of *Confucian* welfare states. After which, the last word belongs to Richard Rose with his case for the re-examination of relations between 'the state, welfare and freedom' in the light of recent experience. It is almost, but not quite, where Professors Klein and Mishra came in.

We are most grateful to the Institute of Contemporary British History for initiating and sponsoring this project, to Peter Caterall in particular for his efforts to ensure the successful running of the day conference and to colleagues attending that event who contributed so much to the quality of discussion and thence to the formulation of this book.

NOTES

1 The conference 'Comparative Social Policy, Trends and Prospects' was held on 17 May 1991 at the Policy Studies Institute, London, before an invited audience. It was sponsored by the Institute of Contemporary British History.
2 In fact Professor Leibfried most generously offered this paper (reproduced in revised and edited version by kind permission of Campus Verlag and Westview Press – see Chapter 7) at short notice, in substitution for one scheduled to be contributed by his colleague Dr Lutz Leisering of the University of Bremen, who was unfortunately prevented from completing his own paper owing to illness.

Part I
On the state of the art

1 O'Goffe's tale

Or what can we learn from the success of the capitalist welfare states?

Rudolf Klein

This paper starts with a puzzle. Looking back on the literature on the welfare state published in the 1970s and the early 1980s (Moran, 1988), there is a striking asymmetry. On the one hand, there are the grim prophecies of crisis – if not worse – threatening the welfare state in capitalist societies. On the other hand, there is the almost total silence about the likely fate of the welfare state in communist societies. Yet if we look around us now, there is a very simple observation to be made. On the one hand, the welfare state in capitalist societies has survived the crisis in remarkably good health. On the other hand, the welfare state in communist societies is going through precisely the same paroxysms of reconstruction as the regimes that created it. It is a contrast which, as I shall argue in this paper, has some important implications for both the practice and theory of comparative social policy studies.

The best starting point for exploring this puzzle is perhaps O'Goffe's tale. In constructing O'Goffe's tale, I have taken the three leading exponents of the neo-Marxist thesis (O'Connor, 1973; Gough, 1979; Offe, 1984) and conflated the main features of their accounts. The result may not be fully fair to any individual member of the trio – and is not intended to be so – but it gives a sense of the logic of their argument. For what distinguished O'Goffe from the myriad of other scholars wringing their hands about the plight of the welfare state at a time of economic turmoil was that he sought to explain these troubles by invoking the nature of *capitalist* states. In O'Goffe's view this was not just a crisis. It was something much more serious: a contradiction. In other words, the difficulties of the welfare state did not just reflect contemporary or evanescent problems of capitalist societies but were inherent in their nature. They were inherent because of the in-built, inescapable conflict between the needs of legitimation, consumption and the demands of capital accumulation. To maintain political legitimacy, the capitalist state had to spend on welfare services and programmes; to maintain the machinery of capitalism, however, it had to promote capital accumulation and ensure profits. And all this was in addition to freeing enough resources for consumption. The development of the welfare state threatened the process of capital accumulation. While the Keynesian Welfare State had for 30 years created the illusion that both objectives of policy could be reconciled in an ever-more prosperous world, the loss of belief both in Keynesian theories of economic management and in the compound arithmetic of growth meant that conflict was inevitable. The conflict could be resolved and the welfare state saved, O'Goffe concluded, only in a new kind of socialist society.

There were important insights in this approach. It was a much-needed antidote to the kind of bland, historicist accounts of the welfare state typical of the hitherto dominant Marmuss school.[1] This tended to present the rise of the welfare state everywhere as an inevitable process: a milestone in the progress of mankind. O'Goffe rightly argued that welfare policies involved conflict about resources, and therefore raised questions about the distribution of power in society. Equally important, he pointed out that welfare policies could not be separated from economic policies, and that both are inevitably shaped by political institutions. In short, O'Goffe concluded, the welfare state could be understood only as the product of economic and political forces: as part of the total social environment.

The impact of O'Goffe's critique was all the greater because it echoed, and in many respects overlapped with, that of Hayman.[2] The New Right also argued that the welfare state would destroy capitalism. The growth of social spending, so the case ran, was undermining work incentives, sapping the ability to invest, creating self-serving welfare bureaucracies and fuelling inflation. Worse still, it was a threat to liberty: the political system was being corrupted (as well as being overloaded) by having to take decisions about the distribution of resources that should be left to the market. Not the least important common element between O'Goffe and Hayman was their shared distrust for the capacity of Western political systems. For very different reasons, they had little faith in politics – seen as a dialogue between groups with different interests but a common concern to solve societal problems – as a way of tackling the difficulties posed by rising social expenditures in times of economic stringency. Indeed, rising social expenditure was seen as a symptom of political failure: democratic politics, it was often argued (Brittan, 1977), generated extravagant public expectations which in turn led to excessive expenditure.

O'Goffe had nothing to say, however, about the welfare state in communist states. Indeed, on his own premises, there was no need to say anything about this. For was not the whole point of his argument that the crisis – indeed contradictions – of the welfare state derived from the very nature of capitalist societies? There was no need to test the premises, even though some of us suggested at the time that it might be a good idea to do so

(Klein, 1979): that communist societies might well have the same dilemmas – such as the conflict between meeting needs and maintaining work incentives and between the demands of capital accumulation and social spending – as capitalist ones. O'Goffe clearly took the premises to be self-evidently true. In fact, the events of the past few years suggest that they were self-evidently wrong: that the same conflicts, contradictions or crises afflicted the communist Welfare States (CWS) as the Keynesian Welfare States (KWS). The real difference lay in the fact that while the capitalist societies of the West were able to cope with the supposedly irreconcilable contradictions, the communist societies of the East collapsed under their weight. While the KWS has emerged virtually intact from the 1980s almost everywhere – a point to which we return below – the CWS is crumbling in the wake of the collapse of the regimes that created it.

A number of implications can be drawn out from O'Goffe's tale. The first is about the logic of political analysis. Before we can make a statement about cause-and-effect in a particular society – or class of societies – we surely have to be able to test it against a counter-factual. Otherwise, we are operating in a solipsistic universe. The point is as obvious as it is frequently neglected. The comparative method is not just a luxury add-on to the study of social policy but an essential component if we are to avoid repeating O'Goffe's blunder in over-predicting the crisis of the welfare state in the West while under-predicting its collapse in the East.

The point can be simply illustrated. Take O'Goffe's assertion about the conflict between the competing claims of political legitimation, capital accumulation and consumption. What evidence is there to support the assumption that this is somehow peculiar or unique to capitalism? None. But if O'Goffe had chosen to search for evidence that such conflict was also apparent in communist regimes, he might well have found it; certainly there are hints that communist regimes used welfare spending as a means of buying legitimacy and popularity (Ferge, 1986) when they failed to deliver the goods of economic prosperity or political acceptability. Indeed, it might quite plausibly be argued (using the O'Goffe line of reasoning) that, in doing so, they damaged their capacity for capital accumulation and further undermined their legitimacy, so creating what proved to be a fatal downward cycle.

But of course it may be argued in O'Goffe's defence that information about social policy in the communist bloc was remarkably scant at the time (as it still is). Therein, however, lies the second implication which can be drawn out from O'Goffe's tale. It suggests the need for self-examination in the social policy community. Why was there so little information in the 1970s and 1980s? And why, as anyone trying to teach comparative social policy soon found, were most of the available studies unsatisfactory in quality? Part of the answer lies, obviously, in the fact that communist regimes did not release accurate data or encourage research; even now it is extraordinarily difficult to establish with precision, for example, what percentage of the national income is spent on health care (or education and the social services) for purposes of comparison. But this is an incomplete answer. Even when there was evidence of the failure of the communist regimes in the welfare field – notably that provided by rising mortality (Wnuk-Lipinsky and Illsley, 1990) – it tended to be neglected in comparative social policy studies.

Similarly, the evidence of parallelisms between capitalist and communist welfare states tended to be overlooked: for example, Wilensky's conclusion (1975) that much the same (non-ideological) factors explained the growth of welfare state spending in capitalist and communist countries. It is therefore difficult to resist the conclusion that the under-prediction of crisis reflected both the linguistic incompetence and ideological predispositions of most of the scholars in the field. There has always been, and continues to be, a serious shortage of scholars in the field equipped with the languages required for the serious study of East European welfare systems. And there is a lingering tendency to use comparative studies as a search for ammunition in domestic political battles: to be able to cite examples of how much better things are done in other (preferably non-capitalist or left-wing) countries.

This is not to imply that O'Goffe was necessarily or invariably uncritical of the welfare state in communist societies. Indeed, some Marxists (Deacon, 1983) argued that the social policies of the Eastern bloc countries were, in themselves, evidence that these countries could not be considered to be fully communist or socialist societies. Despite the limitations of their analysis, dependent as they were on English-language sources, they were able to see the multiple inadequacies of the CWS. The analysis also conceded that, to establish a fully socialist welfare state, there would have to be a 'class struggle' against the political leadership in Eastern Europe. But it crucially stopped short of considering whether a form of economic organisation that rested on the collective ownership of the means of production was compatible with a fully socialist welfare state. Might not the capture of the welfare state by the self-interest of the party bureaucracy represent an inherent, unavoidable contradiction in communist societies? Rather than conceding this point, the Marxist literature sought to argue that some communist regimes had demonstrated that truly socialist social policies were feasible. In Deacon's case, the examples cited were China, Cuba and (incredibly) Mozambique.

In short, the Marxist literature represents the search for a social policy Utopia, i.e. a society where there is no conflict between the self-interest of the welfare state producers and consumers or between competing claims on national resources. The quest for the 'Eldorado banal de tous les vieux marxistes', to adapt Baudelaire, goes on – undiscouraged by the fact that infatuation inevitably leads to disillusion, as successive candidates for the 'Eldorado' turn out to be flawed. While the failures or problems of capitalist societies are seen as being inherent in their very nature, the failures or problems of communist societies are seen only as evidence that they are not truly communist. In the first case, the system is showing its true face; in the second, it is a betrayal of what the system should be like – and therefore no conclusions can be drawn about the model's viability. It is a line of argument which, of course, can never be proved wrong by mere empirical evidence.

To summarise the argument so far, then, the paradox is that the neo-Marxist analysts of the welfare state developed an analytical tool-kit which might well have been quite useful in predicting the impending disintegration of the CWS – but chose not to use it. Instead, they applied their explanatory drill to the KWS, and it broke in their hands. And it broke in their hands precisely because of their assertion that the dilemma of choice was unique to capitalist societies. In doing so, they overlooked the possibility that these societies might have the *political* institutions and resources required to cope with the reconciliation of competing claims and the so-called 'crisis of the welfare state': a rather overblown way of describing the problems of adaptation to new circumstances which faced Western societies in the wake of the global economic crisis of the mid-1970s. In contrast, the communist societies lacked these institutions and resources, which is, of course, why O'Goffe under-predicted the turmoil in the East and over-predicted the crisis in the West. In the next section, we therefore discuss in rather more detail what can be learnt from comparative studies of this success story for the capitalist societies of the West.

FROM CRISIS TO SUCCESS

Although the 1970s spawned a formidable body of literature on the 'crisis of the welfare state' – a phrase which also haunted the early 1980s – the actual story turned out to be one of successful adaptation (Jobert, 1991). The welfare state, on balance, turns out to have discomfited those who were writing its obituary (Ringen, 1987). The contradictions, it turned out, could be managed if not eliminated. If choice between competing claims on increasingly scarce resources could not be avoided – and where, except in Utopia, can it be avoided? – at least Western societies turned out to have the political capacity for dealing with the challenge.

Most important, perhaps, is what has not happened. There has been no crisis of legitimacy in the Western capitalist societies, in sharp contrast to the communist nations of the East. The existing political order has not been challenged. There is little evidence of massive disillusion with the political system. If one of the purposes of social spending is to legitimate the state, as O'Goffe would put it, then it appears to have been achieved. Bismarck's invention, 'conceived of as an essay in practical politics' (King, 1983), has turned out to be a success. The welfare state has helped to maintain the political stability – and probably also the social cohesion – of the Western world.

The achievement is all the more remarkable if we consider that the period of the 'crisis of the welfare state' was also the era of quite exceptional social change and dislocation in Britain and other countries of the West. The nature of the transformation is well known: the move from traditional industry to the service economy (Gershuny, 1978). So is the fact that it was accompanied everywhere by unemployment on a scale which, until the mid-1970s, would have been considered a threat to political stability: no government, so ran the conventional political wisdom of post-1945 Britain, could survive unemployment figures above 500,000 – let alone 1 or 2 million. If the welfare state is conceived of as an instrument for insuring against the risks of change, or as a way of compensating those who bear the social costs (Baldwin, 1990), then again it seems to have earned its keep during these critical years. This is not to assert that the social costs of change were necessarily equitably or fully compensated everywhere; the level of unemployment benefits was one of the casualties of public expenditure retrenchment in many OECD countries (OECD, 1985). It is to argue, however, that – whatever its weaknesses or inequities – the welfare state did succeed in helping to smooth the social and political pains of a dramatic economic transformation.

Nor is there much evidence that social spending was at the expense – as both O'Goffe and the New Right argued – of capital accumulation (Cameron, 1985). The real conflict was between social spending and consumption; hence the famous tax back-lash of the late 1970s. It was this that seemed to vindicate O'Goffe's prophecy. If the accelerating expansion of social spending characteristic of the 1960s and the early 1970s had been maintained, then clearly personal disposable income would have been severely squeezed: public consumption would effectively have replaced private consumption. Extrapolation could easily produce a doom scenario of government bankruptcy and falling personal incomes (Rose and Peters, 1978). In the event, governments did not go bankrupt and, on the whole, personal incomes continued to rise; one of the few countries in which the incomes of the 'middle mass' have failed to rise substantially over the past decade is the United States, a notoriously low welfare spender. For what the predictions of crisis and collapse had overlooked was the institutional resilience of the welfare state and the effect over time of marginal, incremental changes. Nowhere was total welfare state expenditure reduced;

everywhere, however, governments sought ways of reducing the inherited rate of increase.

On the one hand, the welfare state therefore emerged from the 1980s everywhere looking much as it had at the start of the decade. There were no dramatic changes in its institutions, policies and programmes. The welfare state, it turned out, had created a powerful political constituency for its own survival even in countries, like Britain (Hills, 1990) and the United States (Marmor, Mashaw and Harvey, 1990), which had governments ideologically committed to cutting it back. On the other hand, there turned out to be unexpected scope for decelerating the rate of growth in spending. In part, this was achieved by disguising retrenchment as technical change in the method of calculating benefits over time (for example, by decoupling them from movements in earnings); in part, it was done by concentrating economies on those groups with least political power (for example, welfare beneficiaries and the unemployed). On balance, the beneficiaries of the welfare state concentrated in strong, permanent constituencies – like the elderly and the service providers – seem to have emerged remarkably unscathed, while the shifting populations of those at the margins or outside the labour force appear to have done rather worse. The outcome, in fact, is what might be predicted if one sees the welfare state not as an instrument for 'doing good' – let alone for achieving equality – but as both the product and the producer of coalitions of self-interest.

The welfare state also demonstrated, in the 1980s, its capacity for organisational adaptation. In response to economic stringency, it moved to meet some of the criticisms once again common to O'Goffe and the New Right: notably, the criticisms of a self-serving welfare bureaucracy imposing their own preferences on captive consumers. The current reforms of Britain's National Health Service (Day and Klein, 1991) are a case in point, as are the changes in the education system designed to tilt power towards parents, which in part at least inspired the health policies. The NHS changes are more likely to change the balance of power between managers and providers, rather than that between consumers and professionals. But, interestingly, Sweden is currently experimenting with a rather similar set of ideas (Saltman, 1990, and Gould in this volume), if within a totally different ideological framework: there the intention appears to be to see how far it is possible to create choice for health care consumers by forcing public providers to compete for customers. There is, of course, a standard O'Goffe response to such changes. These are seen not as demonstrating a capacity for flexibility or innovation but as evidence that capitalism is trying to re-build the welfare state in its own image; that the welfare state has been saved only at the cost of distorting its real essence by introducing the values of the market place: by commodifying welfare. In short, the prediction of disaster has turned

contention that, given the nature of mankind or of a particular class of society, change will inevitably be either futile or have perverse consequences. What this would suggest is that social policy needs a very different kind of theorising: one that is based not on large and often vacuous generalisations about the nature of capitalist or any other kind of society but on a rigorous analysis of the policy conflicts in particular societies and of the criteria used to justify specific choices (Weale, 1991). Diagnosing 'contradictions', i.e. conflicts, in societies does not get us far. Investigating how different societies tackle those conflicts – their institutional capacity for so doing, the structure of power and the arguments used in the process – is likely to provide far more illumination.

ACKNOWLEDGEMENTS

I am grateful for the comments of all the participants at the conference which gave birth to this book, and for the specific suggestions from Bob Deacon, Nicholas Deakin and Richard Rose.

NOTES

1   Otherwise known as T.H. Marshall and Richard M. Titmuss.
2   Otherwise known as Friedrich A. Hayek and Milton Friedman.

REFERENCES

Baldwin, Peter (1990) *The Politics of Social Solidarity*, Cambridge: Cambridge University Press.
Brittan, Samuel (1977) *The Economic Consequences of Democracy*, London: Temple Smith.
Cameron, David R. (1985) 'Public expenditure and economic performance in international perspective' in Rudolf Klein and Michael O'Higgins (eds) *The Future of Welfare*, Oxford: Basil Blackwell.
Day, Patricia and Klein, Rudolf (1991) 'The British health care experiment', *Health Affairs*.
Deacon, Bob (1983) *Social Policy and Socialism*, London: Pluto Press.
Deutsch, Karl W. (1966) *The Nerves of Government*, New York: The Free Press.
Ferge, Zsuzsa (1986) 'The changing Hungarian social policy' in Else Oyen (ed.) *Comparing Welfare States and their Future*, Aldershot: Gower.
Gershuny, Jonathan (1978) *After Industrial Society?* London: Macmillan.
Gough, Ian (1979) *The Political Economy of the Welfare State*, London: Macmillan.
Hills, John (ed.) (1990) *The State of Welfare*, Oxford: Clarendon Press.
Hirschman, Albert O. (1991) *The Rhetoric of Reaction*, Cambridge, Mass.: The Belknap Press.
Jobert, Bruno (1991) 'La Réstructuration des États Européens', Mimeo, University of Grenoble.

King, Anthony (1983) 'The political consequences of the welfare state' in *Evaluating the Welfare State: Social and Political Perspectives*, London: Academic Press.
Klein, Rudolf (1979) 'Welfare as power', a review of Gough op.cit, *New Society*, 20 September, 632–3.
Marmor, Theodore R., Mashaw, Terry L. and Harvey, Philip L. (1990) *America's Misunderstood welfare state*, New York: Basic Books.
Moran, Michael (1988) 'Crises of the welfare state', *British Journal of Political Science* 18 (3) 397–414.
O'Connor, James (1973) *The Fiscal Crisis of the State*, New York: St Martin's Press.
Offe, Claus (1984) *The Contradictions of the Welfare State*, London: Hutchinson.
Organisation for Economic Co-operation and Development (1985) *Social Expenditure, 1960–1990*, Paris: OECD.
Pfaller, Alfred, Gough, Ian and Therborn, Goran (1991) *Can the welfare state Compete?* London: Macmillan.
Ringen, Stein (1987) *The Possibility of Politics*, Oxford: Clarendon Press.
Rose, Richard and Peters, Guy (1978) *Can Governments Go Bankrupt?* London: Macmillan.
Saltman, Richard B. (1990) 'Competition and reform in the Swedish health system' *The Milbank Quarterly* 68 (4), 597–618.
Weale, Albert (1991) 'Principles, process and policy' in Thomas and Dorothy Wilson (eds) *The State and Social Welfare*, London: Longman.
Wilensky, Harold L. (1975) *The Welfare State and Equality*, Berkeley: University of California Press.
Wnuk-Lipinsky, E. and Illsley, Raymond (1990) 'International comparative analysis: main findings and conclusions' *Social Science and Medicine* 31 (8), 878–89.

2 Social policy in the postmodern world

The welfare state in Europe by comparison with North America

Ramesh Mishra

Since the economic problems of stagflation first surfaced in the early 1970s the state of the welfare state[1] – its present condition and future prospects – has been a matter of almost continuous speculation and debate. The general verdict, as we enter the 1990s, is that the welfare state remains more or less intact. By and large the changes that have occurred have been marginal. The idea of 'irreversibility' or 'maturity' captures this sense of the durability of the welfare state rather well.[2] However, this emphasis on the essential continuity and stability of the institutions of social protection across the 'crisis' decades has resulted, unwittingly perhaps, in a tendency to overlook certain other changes relevant to the unfolding of the welfare state. Essentially these changes are contextual. Ideologically and politically, the welfare state inhabits a very different world today compared with the period before the mid-1970s. It is this changed context and its implications for the welfare state in the West that is the subject matter of this paper. It will be argued that the impact of these changes is likely to be greater on the welfare states of Western Europe than on those of North America.

THE MEANING OF THE WELFARE STATE

As a social system, the post-World War II welfare state derived its meaning and wider historical significance from general theories of social development. Various 'grand narratives' or general interpretations of the development of Western society have sought to capture the 'meaning' or 'essence' of the welfare state by relating it to a wider pattern of social development (George and Wilding, 1976; Mishra, 1981; Room, 1979). Here we shall single out three overarching theories for attention: Marxism, social democracy or democratic transition to socialism, and neo-conservatism. It appears that through the 1980s and early 1990s we are witnessing a decline in the credibility of these theories, especially of their historicist and evolutionary assumptions. Moreover it is a decline which may well be terminal rather than episodic or cyclical. A series of changes – ideological and philosophical, aesthetic and cultural, economic and political – within Western society suggest the emergence of, or at least transition towards, a new situation or condition. A distinctive feature of this situation may be said to be the exhaustion of social utopias. This echoes the notion of 'postmodernity', summed up by an acknowledged philosopher of postmodernity as 'incredulity toward meta narratives' (Lyotard 1984: xxiv).[3]

Meta narratives, or grand narratives, refer to overarching theories or philosophies which promise human emancipation or seek to provide a universal grounding for truth. For postmodern theorists the virtual elimination of the 'communist alternative' in the West following upon the crisis of the Keynesian welfare state offered an example of the 'decline of the unifying and legitimating power of grand narratives of speculation and emancipation' (Lyotard, 1984: 38). Indeed, the dramatic turn of events in the communist world reinforces the notion of the end of an era dominated by grand narratives of emancipation. In sum, the postmodern stage is one where grand narratives have visibly and palpably failed and therefore have very little credibility.

THE END OF UTOPIA

The postmodern notion of the collapse of grand narratives can be translated more concretely as the fading of various historicist and other utopian visions of development in terms of which the post-World War II welfare state has often been understood. Marxism, democratic transition to socialism and neo-conservatism (which differs however in important ways from the other two), are three such overarching perspectives that have been 'tested' in the period following the crisis of the Keynesian welfare state and, in different ways and to differing degrees, found wanting. The predictions and expectations of all three have been belied by history. Welfare capitalism remains more or less intact and shows no sign of collapsing, whether under the weight of inherent contradictions, fiscal crisis or popular revolt of the masses against government 'imposition'. Rather the visions of a pure capitalist society without welfare state and of a socialist society beyond welfare capitalism have both proved illusory. Paradoxically the welfare state, based on the pragmatics of a society that combines a market economy and a democratic polity, remains in place with a measure of stability and autonomy, even while these grand narratives lose credibility as guides to the course of history and to the future of the welfare state.

THE CHANGING IDEOLOGICAL CONTEXT

Marxism

In the Marxist perspective – in terms of both history and scale of values – the welfare state occupied a somewhat lowly position. Since the progression of society from capitalism to socialism was inevitable, the welfare state – a necessary adjunct of advanced capitalism – appeared as little more than a transitory phenomenon destined to disappear with the coming of socialist society.

Welfare capitalism appeared not only as a *transitory* phenomenon in the evolution of Western capitalist society but also as a *contradictory* phenomenon. It was contradictory at the level of both values and institutions. As a hybrid, the welfare state tried to combine socialistic values with an essentially market- and profit-orientated individualistic value system of capitalism. This was one kind of incompatibility. The other was at the institutional level. The privately owned and profit-orientated market economy was not, in the long run, compatible either with a workforce enjoying full employment and social security or with a high level of public expenditure and taxation entailed by the welfare state. In various ways and from somewhat differing perspectives, neo-Marxists such as O'Connor (1973), Habermas (1976), Offe (1984) and Gough (1979) articulated the nature of these deepening contradictions of welfare capitalism in the 1970s and early 1980s and broached the possibility of a system crisis. One scenario was that of a welfare capitalism, which could live neither with nor without social programmes and expenditures, lapsing into a state of 'paralysis' (Offe, 1984: ch. 6). Indeed, at the back of most neo-Marxist analysis has been some expectation of a system crisis that would lead to radical changes, which would usher in socialism and consign the welfare state, at least in the form in which we have known it, to the dustbin of history.

These expectations have proved illusory. Two decades of crises and contradictions of welfare capitalism have shown that revolutionary socialism is not on the agenda. Neither is radical capitalism for that matter.

The mixed economy and the welfare state, albeit somewhat attenuated, remain the reality in Western societies and look like remaining so for the foreseeable future. Capitalism is alive and well, if not positively thriving. The welfare state itself is not doing too badly, all things considered.[4] Thus the two main stipulations of Marxist theory – that the welfare state is transitory and that it is contradictory, i.e. incompatible with a capitalist economy – can no longer claim validity. Indeed, in so far as both the private market economy and electoral democracy have emerged stronger as the key institutions of Western society, the continuation of the mixed economy and the welfare state, in some form or other, seems virtually assured. The collapse of the communist alternative in Eastern Europe and the moves there towards market economy and political democracy suggest a similar pattern of development in ex-communist countries. In sum, as we reach the close of the 1900s, welfare capitalism looks both durable and viable, contradictory or not, while the historicist scenario of a socialist transformation now looks increasingly unrealistic. In short, the idea that history contains within itself the seeds of emancipation from the frustrations and imperfections of a mixed system can no longer be taken seriously.

Democratic transition to Socialism

Unlike Marxism, social democracy has taken a far more favourable view of the welfare state, seeing it largely as a creature of the democratic labour movement and embodying, to a greater or lesser extent, the egalitarian and collectivist values of socialism.[5] Moreover, social policy was not simply a defensive measure – a way of mitigating the rigours of market capitalism by providing some degree of security and equity. It was also a democratic means for advancing society along the road to socialism (Esping-Andersen, 1985; Korpi, 1978; Stephens, 1979). For social democrats have shared with Marxists an historical and evolutionary perspective on socialism.[6] The essential difference between Marxists and social democrats has centred less on the belief in the inevitability of socialism and more on the means of attaining this goal. For Marxists, the capitalist state could not be made to serve the working class and had to be destroyed. For social democrats, on the other hand, the modern democratic state could be a vehicle for the gradual transformation of capitalism through parliamentary and constitutional means (George and Wilding, 1976; Korpi, 1983; Stephens, 1979).

The theory and practice of social democracy have, of course, varied across nations. The idea of a transition to socialism through the developed welfare state seems to have found its highest expression in Swedish socialism. According to Swedish social democrats, transition to socialism takes place through a series of stages (Korpi, 1978: 85; Olsson, 1990: 113). The first stage is that of political democracy. The workers win the struggle for franchise and the right to form unions and other associations. With mass democracy, the organisation of trade unions and the rise of labour parties comes the second stage, that of social democracy and the welfare state. In this stage production still remains in the hands of capital but distribution begins to be socialized and labour is able to put some restraints on capital. This period represents an 'historic compromise' between labour and capital in which economic growth allows a positive-sum rather than a zero-sum game to be played. Both capitalism and the working class go through a process of maturation which prepares society for the next stage, namely that of economic democracy (Korpi, 1978: 320). According to prominent Swedish social scientists such as Korpi, this stage was reached in Sweden by the early 1970s. The historic compromise had come to an end and labour was prepared for the next stage (Korpi, 1983: ch. 10; Pontusson, 1984). As a first step towards the next stage, i.e. economic democracy, the Swedish labour movement proposed the so-called wage-earners' funds (Korpi, 1983: 232–4).

These funds proved a contentious measure for the social democratic movement and even more so for the country at large. A form of wage-earners' fund was enacted in 1983 but represented a considerably watered down version of what was intended initially (Ahlen 1989: 189–90, 192; Heclo and Madsden 1987: ch. 6; also Gould in this volume). While it may be too early to pronounce on the fate of 'economic democracy' in general and wage-earners' funds in particular, the experience so far does not suggest that these funds can be seen as having initiated the advance towards economic democracy (Pontusson, 1987: 24). Moreover, social democracy outside Sweden seems to have no ideas or proposals for a transition towards socialism.

While social democratic governments, by and large, have been among the staunch defenders of the welfare state, it would be presumptuous to suggest that this has anything to do with transition to socialism. Rather, the evidence suggests a pragmatic defence of the welfare state. Indeed, far from moving toward socialism, most social democratic governments have taken steps to reduce the burden of taxation, especially on higher incomes, have trimmed social expenditures in order to reduce deficit and, at best, have tried to hold the line on rising unemployment (see Gould in this volume; Mishra, 1990: ch. 3; Walters, 1985: 366–8). Transition to socialism is nowhere on the agenda; strengthening the capitalist market economy is everywhere on the agenda. In short, under social democratic regimes as elsewhere, the welfare state is proving to be little more than a junior partner within the enterprise of welfare capitalism dominated by a market economy and the ethos of private consumption.

The neo-conservatives

The most recent 'grand narrative' concerned with the welfare state is that of neo-conservatism (Friedman and Friedman, 1980; Gilder, 1982; King, 1987; Steinfels, 1979). This theory of voluntarism, market and the minimal state, which combines elements of explanation with strong prescription, has, of course, been the most vociferous since the days of stagflation and the crisis of the welfare state in the mid-1970s. At that time it launched a fierce attack on the welfare state, alleging that it was the source of all our economic ills. Indeed, the more strident elements of the New Right expected a citizens' revolt against big government and taxation resulting in a massive retrenchment, if not the demise, of the welfare state (Friedman and Friedman, 1980: ch. 10). Not a socialist revolution but a neo-conservative *counter*-revolution was to liberate the masses from the tyranny of the state. In this Utopia of the right there would be only individuals, markets, voluntary associations and charities. State welfare programmes would be reduced to the very minimum, so that the Keynesian welfare state would be no more than a memory of our past follies.

It is of course against the heady rhetoric of the New Right that leftist thinkers such as Offe (1984), Piven and Cloward (1985) and Therborn (1984) counterposed the idea of the irreversibility of the welfare state. Now, nearly 20 years after the stagflation crisis of welfare capitalism and a decade of neo-conservative regimes in countries such as the UK and the USA, we cannot say that mainstream social programmes have been substantially retrenched anywhere (Brown, 1988; Friedmann *et al.*, 1987). The Utopia of the right – a capitalism without the welfare state – remains a fantasy.

True, welfare states everywhere have been shrinking somewhat and they have done so rather more under neo-conservatives. Full employment too, as understood in the Keynesian era, is a thing of the past. Moreover, the influence of neo-conservative ideas and policies on the future development of the welfare state is not to be underestimated (Mishra, 1990: ch. 2). Nonetheless, the mixed economy and especially substantial state programmes of social welfare look like being around for the foreseeable future. In this context, it is important to remember that neo-conservatives, in the manner of Marxists, have emphasised the incompatibility of a market economy with state regulation and substantial social welfare. In order to revive growth, they argued that taxes had to be lowered, social expenditures slashed, full employment abandoned and the economy deregulated.

In the light of a quarter-century of spectacular economic growth since World War II under the aegis of a mixed economy, full employment and burgeoning social expenditure, the thesis of incompatibility carried a heavy charge of ideology. The experience since the mid-1970s confirms the observation of many social scientists and political economists: namely that the size of the public sector or the level of social expenditure *per se* had little to do with economic growth and that there was nothing inherently dysfunctional about the mixed economy and welfare capitalism (Cameron, 1982; Kuttner, 1984). Indeed, the argument could as well go the other way, i.e. that it was a vigorous hybrid rather than a contradictory mixture. Be that as it may, the mixed economy of welfare capitalism remains the reality in Western countries and, while the ingredients of the mix may have changed somewhat and might change further, there is no reason to believe that welfare capitalism is likely to give way to laissez-faire capitalism.

The three perspectives on the welfare state reviewed above have one thing in common: in different ways all see the hybrid of welfare capitalism as a transient phenomenon. The dislocations of the Keynesian welfare state in the mid-1970s provided the occasion for all three to envision the transcendence of the mixed economy and the welfare state. It now appears that the development of Western society and the future of the welfare state envisioned in these grand scenarios are quite out of line with the somewhat prosaic reality of the persistence of social programmes and expenditures in all Western countries. True, it is the scenarios of the left that have carried a heavy charge of historicist and evolutionary assumptions – assumptions whose validity is seriously in question. By contrast, the utopia of the right has been largely normative and prescriptive rather than historicist. All the same, the persistence of the hybrid of welfare capitalism, at variance with the predictions or prescriptions of both the left and the right, appears to confirm the postmodern notion of a decline in the credibility of historicism and social Utopias.

THE POLITICAL ECONOMY OF POSTMODERNISM

End of full employment

Far from the development of economic democracy which would succeed the welfare state, what we are witnessing is a trend towards the internationalisation of capital which makes it more difficult for the nation-state to control the economy effectively (Drache and Gertler, 1991; Keane and Owens, 1986; Lash and Urry, 1987). A major development of the last two decades has been the growing trend towards the transnational production of goods. National and multinational companies have been moving some or all of their production processes out of high-wage economies into countries with low labour costs, e.g. the Third World. Production processes are being split more and more into sub-processes that may be carried out anywhere in the world. Moreover, new technologies have been substituting capital for labour, resulting in dramatic increases in productivity but not in jobs (Keane and Owens, 1986:20–1; Therborn, 1986:38–9).

The implications for full employment (at a reasonable wage) are not difficult to imagine. The end of fixed exchange rates of currencies since the early 1970s, the greater volume of international free trade and transnational movements of money and capital have combined to create a situation of much greater volatility and instability compared with the 1950s and 1960s. The precise ways in which these phenomena impinge on the welfare state is not clear. But at the very least, it would seem that global movement of money and capital together with changes in technology and methods of production are making it more difficult for the nation-state to influence the economy and to ensure full employment.

This is not to claim that development is driven simply by economic or technological change. As Therborn has shown, for example, policies and politics do matter. Regimes were able to maintain full or near-full employment in the decade after the OPEC price shock if they had an institutionalized commitment to do so (Therborn, 1986: 23). Therborn draws attention to the fact that regimes have responded in quite diverse ways to the problems faced by the Keynesian welfare state and the new international division of labour (Therborn, 1986: 23). However, this emphasis on policy choice does not in any way contradict the notion that, compared with the preceding decades, Western economies have found it far more difficult to maintain full employment since the early 1970s. From this viewpoint it could be argued that the favourable conjunction of factors that made full employment rather easy to attain in the quarter-century or so after the war has definitely passed away. As many commentators have pointed out, Keynesian demand management policies perhaps played a smaller part in maintaining high levels of employment than is generally believed (Keane and Owens, 1986: 58).

A fortuitous combination of factors resulted in high and sustained demand for labour in Western industrial economies down to the early 1970s. The post-World War II welfare state was a beneficiary of this conjuncture. The world has moved on and we are now in a different international economic environment where it has become far more difficult to ensure that everyone who wants a job can find one. Given the changes in the international division of labour and the globalisation of capital, it appears that the welfare state of the post-WWII era, with full employment as one of its major ingredients, has now passed into history. Regimes no doubt differ in their approach to unemployment. Nonetheless it seems increasingly likely that the problem of work and adequate income will have to be tackled in ways other than those associated with the Keynesian welfare state, such as some form of income guarantee (Drache and Gertler, 1991: 21; Keane and Owens, 1986: 175–6).

Tripartism in decline

A significant development of the 1980s seems to be the decline of neo-corporatism or tripartism as a mode of conflict management (Lash and Urry, 1987: ch. 8; Schmitter, 1989). Countries such as Sweden and Austria were able to maintain high levels of employment and social programmes and expenditures largely owing to the consensus and cooperation around economic policies between organised labour and business. In particular, centralised wage negotiation and wage moderation played an important part in keeping inflation under control and making full employment and economic growth possible (Mishra, 1990: ch. 3; Martin, 1986: 173–4, 201–5). Indeed, after the weakening of Keynesian welfare capitalism in countries such as Britain, it looked for a time as if the 'integrated welfare state' typical of social corporatist countries might provide a viable alternative to neo-conservative policies of monetarism, unemployment, decentralised wage bargaining and welfare cutbacks (Banting, 1986; Mishra, 1984: ch. 4). However, by now it is clear that the conditions which made a neo-corporatist approach to the economic management of welfare capitalism feasible have weakened considerably. In part it is a matter of the cross-national mobility of capital and production. The trends noted earlier in this regard have strengthened the hands of capital against labour very considerably – e.g. via the threat of investing abroad – and have at the same time made it more difficult to strike a bargain with national capital, whose interests are no longer confined to the nation-state. At the same time, the situation of the labour force has been changing in a way that is also weakening tripartism (Lash and Urry, 1987: ch. 8; Schmitter, 1989). For instance:

1   The prospect of sustained economic growth, typical of the 1960s and early 1970s, was highly conducive to voluntary wage restraint on the part of workers. Such expectations are no longer realistic.
2   Employers, for their part, supported tripartism in conditions of full employment and labour scarcity in order to promote wage restraint, technological change and industrial peace. With the end of full employment and the weakening of the unions, employers now find market-based solutions to these problems more attractive.
3   The growing heterogeneity of the labour force is also helping to unravel tripartism. The core of blue-collar workers employed in the private sector formed the mainstay of the identity and solidarity of the centralised trade union movement and national-level bargaining. These workers are now a declining section of the labour force. Partly through the growth of white-collar jobs and partly through the growth of the public sector, itself a product of the welfare state, important cleavages have opened up within the union movement. Increasingly, the unity and solidarity of labour as a 'social partner' have been weakened, resulting in the trend towards sectional bargaining and the erosion of a voluntary incomes policy. Sweden, in many ways a model country in respect of corporatism until recently, shows these trends quite well (see Gould in this volume; Ahlen, 1989; Lash and Urry, 1987: ch. 8). In short, the neo-corporatist defence of the welfare state looks a less viable option.

From class politics to plural politics

Although the importance of class – whether seen in socioeconomic terms or as rooted in the ownership of means of production – for contemporary politics cannot be underestimated, action based on other identities and interests seems to be relativising class politics. Thus feminist and ethnic interests, ecological movements, community activism and other grassroots organisations – in brief, 'new' social movements – cut across class lines. Moreover their approach to politics and social change often differs from that of organised labour and established political parties (Dalton *et al.*, 1990; Offe, 1985). We seem to be witnessing the emergence of interest groups critical of the centralised, statist and bureaucratic forms of social policy associated with the Keynesian welfare state.

While it is important not to exaggerate the significance of the trend toward plural politics, the trend seems to conform to the idea of postmodernists, namely that 'local narratives' tend to replace 'grand narratives'. As each group discovers through the political process that, for example, the claim of a particular movement (e.g. labour) to stand for universal emancipation (e.g. of gender and race) cannot be entertained, political interests are invariably fragmented. The exact nature and scope of the relativisation of class politics, the growth of interests around other identities and, in particular, the resulting implications for the politics of the welfare state remain for the moment unclear (Lash and Urry, 1987: 209–31; Olofsson, 1988). We may be witnessing the growth of important new interests, based for example on gender and age, concerned with public welfare policies. For these social groups, social welfare may have a great deal of importance but of a rather specific kind. In short, we may find that, while the constituency for the welfare state grows wider and more varied, the values and interests that animate constituent groups may have less to do with the general distributive concerns typical of the labour movement. In sum, given the validity of the ideological and other changes sketched earlier in the paper, it is likely that the labour movement will be less influential in shaping the nature of welfare politics in the future. Even so, this is not to deny the salience of class for politics nor is it to question the capability of social democracy of leading the struggle for security, equity and social justice on behalf of groups other than the working class.

COMPARING NORTH AMERICA AND WESTERN EUROPE

We have identified a number of significant trends and developments – conveniently labelled as 'postmodern' – and considered their implications for the welfare state in a general way. Yet in reality welfare states and their socio-political contexts vary from one country to another and from one part of the world to another. It is therefore to be expected that the implications of postmodernity will vary likewise. It will be argued that (i) North American developments have differed in significant ways from those of Western Europe in the post-World War II era (which admittedly is not saying anything new); (ii) postmodern developments are likely to have a greater impact on West European welfare states; and (iii) these developments are likely to bring the political economy (though not necessarily the social policy) of European welfare states somewhat closer to that of North America.[7]

However, before we consider the reasoning and evidence for such a 'one-way' convergence towards the North American pattern, it is necessary to clarify what we mean by 'North American' and 'West European' welfare states. Although all 'actually existing' welfare states are unique, it is nonetheless possible to single out features that are common to a group of welfare states and that distinguish this group from others. In this sense, then, despite important differences within North America, i.e. between Canada and the United States, and even more pronounced differences among West European countries, it is possible to identify certain features characteristic of North America and others more characteristic of Western Europe. It is in this sense that we shall highlight features common to such European countries as the UK, Germany, Austria and Sweden and contrast them with those common to Canada and the United States.[8] In short, we shall accentuate intra-region similarity while at the same time accentuating *inter-region* dissimilarity. We consider below the implications of postmodernity in the context of these ideal-typical differences between the two regions of North America and Western Europe.

Decline of Utopia

The ideas of evolution and historicism, associated above all with the left, have had a great deal of purchase in Europe. They have found institutional expression in the communist and social democratic parties which have had close ties with trade unions and other working class organisations. Of particular relevance to the post-WWII era has been the idea of a gradual transition to socialism under the auspices of the labour movement and through parliamentary means. As argued earlier (p. 21 above), in the context of a democratic advance towards socialism the welfare state appeared as both a necessary and a transitory phenomenon. The collectivism and egalitarianism associated with the welfare state became invested with an aura of historical inevitability in the course of the presumed evolution towards socialism. It is this historical utopia which seems to have lost credibility in recent times. True, the expectations of the right, namely that a capitalist market society purged of state welfare might emerge in the West, have also proved illusory. But, in so far as the utopia of the right has been primarily normative and prescriptive rather than historicist and evolutionary in nature, it has suffered rather less from recent developments. Moreover, the fall of communism and the apparent impasse of socialism enable neo-conservatives to see these developments as a vindication of some of their principal tenets.

It is no secret that socialism – both as ideology and as politics – has had far less influence in North America. 'Why is there no socialism in the United States?' is a question that was asked by Sombart (1976) as far back as 1905 and it has been a matter of speculation ever since. Be that as it may, neither the goal of socialism nor the idea of the working class as the prime agent of historical change can be said to have had much relevance in the United States, especially since World War II (Edsall, 1984:chs 1, 4; Piven and Cloward, 1985: ch. 6). True, the Democratic Party has been far more supportive of the welfare state than the Republican Party, having presided over the two major expansionary phases – the New Deal in the 1930s and the Great Society programmes of the 1960s. But this has little to do with the idea of transition to socialism. Unlike most capitalist countries, the United States never developed a social democratic party with the vision of an alternative society. Moreover, the proportion of the workforce unionised in the United States has been far lower than in Western Europe and organised labour has been a good deal less cohesive and centralised (Table 2.1). In short, in the United States the welfare state has never formed part of an agenda of transition to socialism.

The situation in Canada has differed somewhat in this respect. Canada has had a higher level of union membership and, unlike the United States, shows little sign of a decline in membership. It also boasts a social democratic party (NDP). Although the NDP has never managed to receive more than about a fifth of the popular vote, and therefore never come anywhere near forming the government, it has been and remains a considerable presence in Canadian politics (Thornburn, 1985: 30–5, 349). It has formed the government in a number of provinces (chalking up an impressive victory in the rich and populous province of Ontario recently) and, as a party which has on occasions held the balance of power between the two major national parties, has influenced the development of social programmes. All the same, the NDP and the Canadian labour movement as a whole have been rather pragmatic. The party's goals have been Keynesian and orientated towards welfare. The evolutionary and historicist assumptions of the European left have found only a pale echo within the Canadian labour movement (Brodie and Jenson, 1988: 1–4, 272–80).

Thus taking Canada and the United States together, we can say that in North America the idea of the welfare state as a milestone in the journey to

Table 2.1 Union membership and organisational unity of labour, 1965–80

	Membership[a]		Cohesion[b]	Centralization[c]
North America:				
Canada	27	(39)	0.4	0.0
United States	21	(25)	0.4	0.0
Western Europe:				
Austria	50	(58)	1.0	0.8
Britain	45	(54)	0.4	0.3
Germany (West)	32	(33)	0.8	0.2
Sweden	70	(85)	0.8	0.7

[a]   Union membership as a percentage of labour force. Figures in parenthesis are for 1980s
    and are based on percentage of wage and salary earners.
[b]   Higher score (maximum 1.0) denotes greater organizational unity.
[c]   Higher score (maximum 1.0) denotes greater centralization of collective bargaining.

Source: Cameron (1984: 164–5) for membership, cohesion and centralisation, 1965–80.
Therborn (1984: 11) for union membership in 1980.

socialism has had far less significance than in Western Europe. Recent ideological changes associated with 'postmodernity' therefore have much less significance for North America. To simplify in the extreme, we could say that, in this sense, North America has been 'postmodern'*avant la lettre* (Pierson, 1990).

The end of full employment

The commitment to full employment was a prominent feature of the leading welfare states of Western Europe during the early post-World War II decades. This commitment varied, in strength and consistency, from one welfare state regime to another and from one country to another (Apple, 1980). But it cannot be denied that it was an important element in the so-called post-war 'settlement' in the conflict between capital and labour. The end of full employment – at first in practice and later virtually as a policy commitment – is one of the major changes in the welfare states of Western Europe since the economic crisis of the mid-1970s. While some regimes have struggled valiantly to maintain full employment, overall the globalisation of the economy, the growth of new ('post-Fordist') methods of production, freer trade between nations and the mobility of capital have meant acquiescing in a higher rate of unemployment. With a few exceptions, the full-employment welfare state of the Keynesian era is now history (see Figure 2.1).

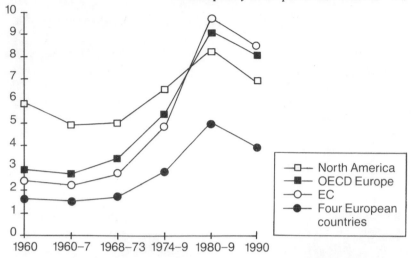

Figure 2.1 Rates of unemployment in Europe and North America, 1960–90.

In contrast with the advanced West European countries, North America never really subscribed to a policy of full employment. In the reconstruction period after WWII the United States rejected the goal of full employment, while Canada's commitment was far weaker than, e.g. that of Britain (Apple, 1980: 10–18). Not surprisingly, unemployment rates in the United States and Canada have been much higher than those in Western Europe (Figure 2.1). Since the mid-1970s however, as Figure 2.1 shows, European rates have drawn closer to, and in the 1980s even exceeded, those of North America. True the *average* unemployment rate for our four 'sample' countries remains well below that of North America's, but at a level three times that of their average for 1960s. Thus the end of full employment as an aspect of the welfare state has greater significance for Western Europe than it has for North America.

Tripartism in decline

Not all West European countries developed structures of decision-making and bargaining which involve peak associations of business and labour together with the state (Banting, 1986; Lehmbruch, 1982). Moreover, in only a few countries, notably Austria and Sweden, have these bipartite or tripartite structures been in place for a relatively long period of time. Nonetheless, all four countries in our 'sample' of European welfare states (Britain, West Germany, Austria and Sweden) have been involved, to a greater or lesser extent and in some form or another, with tripartism (Lehmbruch, 1982; Panitch, 1986).

By contrast tripartism has been virtually absent from North America. The reasons for this need not concern us here (Banting, 1986; Salisbury, 1979; Wilson, 1982). Suffice to say that the absence of such conditions as full employment, a strong and centralised labour movement and a social democratic government are among the factors which have inhibited the development of tripartism in North America. A full-employment welfare state, in which wage moderation is traded off against full employment and social welfare through a form of 'societal bargaining' among social partners, has never been a feature of North America. Although in both the United States and Canada moves towards tripartism were made occasionally they did not amount to much (Fournier, 1986; Wilson, 1982:229). Monetarism coupled with state directives (e.g. statutory incomes policies and back-to-work legislation in Canada, or outright repression, e.g. the sacking of air traffic controllers, in the United States) has been used to control wages and inflation (Edsall, 1984: 161; Moody, 1987; Panitch and Swartz, 1985). The decline of corporatism and the fragmentation of organised labour as a force have far greater significance for Western Europe than for North America.

From class politics to plural politics

Politics (especially lower-class political behaviour) in North America has been far less orientated towards class than in West Europe (Brodie and Jenson, 1988: ch. 1; Edsall, 1984:197; Korpi, 1983:35). As we have noted already, organised labour and social democracy have neither of them been a strong feature. Moreover, since tripartism has never been a feature of North American societies, its recent decline means correspondingly little. Interest groups of various kinds as well as social movements, especially in the United States, have played a more important part in the development of the welfare state (Piven and Cloward, 1985: 163–8; Weir *et al.*, 1988: 15–16). In the United States, for instance, social struggles centred on race have been important in the post-WWII years. As in Europe, new social movements concerned with gender and environment-related and other issues have also developed in North America but often overlapping with the older social movements (Gelb, 1990; Rucht, 1990). Thus in the United States it is not easy to distinguish the one from the other. Hence, by comparison with their European counterparts, scholars and activists in the United States seem 'much less familiar' with the concept of 'new social movements' and are even 'baffled when confronted with it' (Rucht, 1990: 157).

As far as the welfare state is concerned, working-class politics, dominant in the 1950s and 1960s, especially in Europe, has increasingly been challenged and to some extent bypassed by politics based on gender, race and age (Dalton, *et al.*, 1990; Lash and Urry, 1987: 209–31). If the women's movement is a phenomenon common to most advanced countries (for all that its nature and style vary a good deal), the same cannot be said of social activism associated with race and especially age. It is once again in the United States that age-related interest groups have played an important part in the defence of social welfare, e.g. against the Reagan cutbacks in social security (Pratt, 1983). In Canada, too, recent years have seen a good deal of activity centred on culture and ethnicity (French Canadians, native Indian population) as well as on gender (Burt, 1990; Milne, 1990). In so far as the trend in Europe is towards a relative decline of working-class politics and the growth of plural politics, related to social movements and organised interests other than labour, the change seems to be towards the North American pattern.

CONCLUSION

It has been argued that important changes – economic, political and ideological, but above all ideological – have been taking place affecting the wider societal context of the welfare state. Seemingly we are witnessing the end of utopia. Grand narratives concerned with social development and historical evolution, some of which date back to the eighteenth and nineteenth centuries, have suffered a serious lack of credibility. History can no longer be seen as having a particular direction. Clearly what we are witnessing is not the end of 'history' as such but rather the demise of historicist and evolutionist narratives and expectations (Descombes, 1980: chs 4, 6; Fukuyama, 1989).

But, it might be argued, there is a sense of *déjà vu* about all this. Did not the 'end of ideology' thesis in the late 1950s and early 1960s suggest developments of this kind (Bell, 1960; Kerr *et al.*, 1960; Lipset, 1960: ch. xiii)? True, there are some parallels with that definition of the situation. But there are also important differences to be noted. The end of ideology thesis assumed a growing consensus about the nature of major social institutions in advanced industrial society, including the welfare state. Moreover, it saw this consensus as virtually a product of functional necessities inherent in the very nature of modern industrial societies. Technological determinants, together with a set of values and attitudes characteristic of modernity, were seen as the most important factors in shaping the social structure. In this equation neither the capitalist economy nor the liberal polity counted for much. Indeed, capitalism – private ownership of capital and market economy – itself appeared as an outmoded concept, in that the modern industrial economy was seen as having moved beyond capitalist/socialist distinctions based on ownership, market and the like. The managed and regulated mixed economy of 'pluralistic industrialism' was believed to have transcended those antinomies (Kerr *et al.*, 1960: ch.8; see also Galbraith, 1967; Mishra, 1981: ch. 3). In sharp contrast to this thesis, the collapse of communism in Eastern Europe has underlined the importance of the distinction between market and command economies as well as between dictatorships and liberal democracies. It has also shown the poverty of the theory of technological determinism.

Yet another aspect of the end of ideology thesis was the idea that a social science – positivistic and modelled on the natural sciences – was coming of age and would be able to provide neat technicist solutions to social problems such as crime and poverty. Thus, parallel with the idea of a consensus over social arrangements was the notion of a growing consensus about the nature of social knowledge and *its* validation (Mishra, 1981: ch. 1). It is evident from the tenets of postmodernity presented above that its definition of the situation differs in important ways from that of the end of ideology perspective. Postmodernity rejects the possibility of a general consensus, whether about knowledge and its validation or about the role of reason in human emancipation (Boyne and Rattansi, 1990:16–18). The idea that grand narratives are being replaced by 'local narratives' suggests a continuing diversity and plurality of values, beliefs and interests – rather than an imminent consensus – in the postmodern society. In short, what is implied is more akin to the end of *utopia* than of *ideology*. If there are no privileged agencies, beliefs or values in history and no grounds for a consensus, then it is the interplay of a diversity of beliefs, values and interests that defines the postmodern situation (Boyne and Rattansi, 1990:17–19, 39; Lyotard, 1984:65–6).

As far as the welfare state is concerned it means that global formulations which saw the welfare state as transient and as likely to be absorbed and transformed into socialism or else dismantled with a return to good sense and a pure market society or again as simply a set of consensual institutions – an inevitable concomitant of advanced industrialism – can no longer be seen as credible. However, the collapse of grand narratives does not mean that the normative and analytical elements underlying these various perspectives have also lost their relevance. Political and social ideologies of a *relative* kind associated with particular group interests and/or diverse values such as equality, liberty, human rights, ecological responsibility, social justice and the like will continue to lend colour and drama to social choice. Conflict and compromise centred on these diverse values and interests will remain the stuff of social policy. Thus national or regional variations in the interplay of institutional legacy, political ideology and group interests will continue to offer rich material for the comparative study of social policy (George and

Wilding, 1976; Esping-Andersen, 1990). But this is a far cry from the historicist and evolutionary views of social policy development influential in earlier decades.

The seismic changes taking place in Eastern Europe and the USSR would seem to confirm the postmodern thesis. The collapse of communist regimes, and the struggle to create a market economy and a liberal polity in these societies, furnishes a dramatic example of a turning away from utopia – from the totalising narratives of development and emancipation (see Deacon in this volume). In so far as the ex-communist societies are aiming at a social order with a market economy and a liberal polity (though as societies-in-transition they of course encounter special problems), their situation is no different in principle from that of the Western democracies.

If, as this paper has suggested, the age of utopia is over and in both the East and West we are in a post-utopian phase, then another conclusion follows: the post-World War II 'welfare state' as a social formation has also passed into history. For the welfare state, or welfare capitalism if you will, represented a 'middle way' between the extremes of laissez-faire capitalism and paternalistic communism. In this sense the post-World War II welfare state can also be seen as a byproduct of the Cold War, a response on the part of Western capitalism to the challenge of communism. Communism offered employment for all within a system of command economy and polity; the welfare state promised the same but within the confines of a free society. Communism promised to take care of the basic needs of the population through a system of free, collective consumption which also expressed the classless nature of communist society. The welfare state promised to do the same through its universal services which also signified solidarity and decommodification. Communism promised an end to poverty and to create plenty for all; the welfare state offered the same through a market economy suitably equipped with social security and other anti-poverty measures. The welfare state, in short, was the West's answer to the challenge of communism as an alternative social order. Now with the collapse of communism *and* the fading of the neo-conservative vision of a return to laissez-faire capitalism, the 'middle way' itself disappears as the 'left' and the 'right' alternatives, in a strong sense, also disappear.

Moreover, if there is one major implication of postmodernity for welfare it is that the Dionysian spirit of innovation, change and material progress embodied in the market economy has emerged as pre-eminent in the postmodern world.

The Apollonian spirit embodied in social welfare, no matter how expansive, seems destined to remain a subsidiary element, one which in the broadest sense must harmonise with the imperatives of the economy. Paraphrasing Marxism, therefore, one might say that the economy has indeed emerged as the determinant in the last instance, albeit in somewhat unforeseen ways. Further, the pre-eminence of the 'economic' sphere means that not only full employment but also universality can no longer be seen as sacrosanct in the postmodern world. Given that the highest values of the dominant elites and the large part of the masses centre on consumerism, free enterprise and economic growth (with the implied acceptance of vast inequalities as legitimate), it is unlikely that universality as a principle of social provision can survive for long. And once we bid farewell to full employment as well as to universality, the 'welfare state' as a distinct phase in the evolution of social policy in the West will have come to an end. Social policy, in its manifold variation across 'capitalist' countries, will remain a feature of the postmodern age, but the post-war 'welfare state' as a distinct expression of social policy – a 'settlement' between capital and labour in the West as a response to the challenge of radical socialism – will have passed into history.

In any case, in this post-utopian and postmodern situation, social policy emerges more clearly as a relatively autonomous sphere of action which questions, modifies as well as complements the 'economic' mode of being. Paradoxically, and in keeping with the tenets of postmodernity itself, social policy divested of utopian and historicist elements may become truer to itself as an arena for the interplay of the micro-politics of values and interests.

NOTES

1 The term 'welfare state', used in a wide variety of ways, generally refers to the social welfare activities of the state. Here it refers to government commitment and effort in Western industrial countries to maintain a decent minimum standard of living through a high level of employment, general social programmes and anti-poverty measures. For a fuller discussion of the problem of definition, see Mishra (1984: ch. 1) and Mishra (1990: 18–9, 123–4).

2 Social scientists of diverse ideological persuasion seem to share the view that, despite the rhetoric of dismantling and retrenching the welfare state, major social programmes and levels of social expenditures in most Western industrial countries remain largely intact. See, e.g. Heclo (1981), Legrand and Winter (1987), Offe (1984), Piven and Cloward (1985: ch. 6), Therborn and Roebroek (1986). See Mishra (1990: 32–43) for a critique of the 'irreversibility' thesis.

3 There is a burgeoning literature on postmodernity. For a perceptive book length introduction see Boyne and Rattansi (1990). For a brief overview, and an application of the idea to planning, see Simonsen (1990).

4 Although full employment has been abandoned in most Western countries, universal social programmes and expenditures have not been reduced very much even in the UK and the USA. See the various country studies in Brown (1988) and Friedmann *et al.* (1987).

5 For an early post-war discussion, see Crosland (1956). For more recent views, see George and Wilding (1976: ch. 4), Esping-Andersen (1985: ch. 5), Korpi (1983) and Stephens (1979).

6 The term 'social democracy' is used here in the broader European (Continental) sense of the term. The Anglo-Saxon usage suggests a position midway between liberalism and democratic socialism. Social democratic politics of course includes the left tendency – concerned with a democratic but radical transformation of capitalism – as well as the right tendency – content with a form of capitalism with a human face. However, even the most deradicalised social democratic movement has tended to keep alive the myth of socialism and has projected the vision of a relatively different society as a distant but attainable goal while in practice accommodating to capitalism. It is in such a context that the welfare state has come to be seen as a staging post in a long journey.

7 The convergence in question refers to unemployment and some of the other contextual features of the welfare state only. This does not rule out change in the opposite direction in respect of other aspects of the welfare state and social policy. For example, it seems very likely that the United States will institute some form of national health insurance in the near future, a move in the West European direction.

8 Clearly the choice of European countries is biased in favour of full employment welfare states with the history of a strong to medium association with tripartite (corporatist) forms of policy-making at least until the late 1970s. While these countries (and the features they exemplify) can in no way be seen as 'representative of West Europe', they may be seen as typifying one of the major tendencies in post-WWII Western Europe.

REFERENCES

Ahlen, K. (1989) 'Swedish collective bargaining under pressure', *British Journal of Industrial Relations* 27 (3).

Apple, N. (1980) 'The rise and fall of full employment capitalism', *Studies in Political Economy*, No. 4.

Banting, K. (1986) 'The state and economic interests: an introduction' in K. Banting (ed.) *The State and Economic Interests*, Toronto: University of Toronto Press.

Bell, D. (1960) *The End of Ideology*, New York: The Free Press.

Boyne, R. and Rattansi, A. (1990) *Postmodernism and Society*, London: Macmillan.

Brodie, J. and Jenson, J. (1988) *Crisis, Challenge and Change: Party and Class in Canada Revisited*, Ottawa: Carleton University Press.

Brown, M.K. (ed.) (1988) *Remaking the Welfare State*, Philadelphia: Temple University Press.

Burt, S. (1990) 'Rethinking Canadian politics: The impact of gender' in M.S. Whittington and G. Williams (eds) *Canadian Politics in the 1990s*, Scarborough: Nelson Canada.

Cameron, D.R. (1982) 'On the limits of public economy'. *The Annals of the American Academy of Political and Social Science*, Beverly Hills and London: Sage.

—— (1984) 'Social democracy, corporatism, labour quiescence, and the representation of economic interest in advanced capitalist society' in

J.H. Goldthorpe (ed.) *Order and Conflict in Contemporary Capitalism*, Oxford: Clarendon Press.

Crosland, C.A.R. (1956) *The Future of Socialism*, London: Cape.

Dalton, R.J., Kuechler, M., Burklin, W. (1990) 'The challenge of new movements' in R.J. Dalton and M. Kuechler (eds) *Challenging the Political Order*, New York: Oxford University Press.

Descombes, V. (1980) *Modern French Philosophy*, Cambridge: Cambridge University Press.

Drache, D. and Gertler, M.S. (1991) 'The world economy and the nation-state' in D. Drache and M.S. Gertler (eds) *The New Era of Global Competition*, Montreal and Kingston: McGill–Queen's University Press.

Edsall, T.B. (1984) *The New Politics of Inequality*, New York: W.W. Norton & Co.

Esping-Andersen, G. (1985) *Politics Against Markets*, Princeton, NJ: Princeton University Press.

—— (1990) *The Three Worlds of Welfare Capitalism*, Princeton, NJ: Princeton University Press.

Fournier, P. (1986) 'Consensus building in Canada' in K. G. Banting (ed.) *The State and Economic Interests*, Toronto: University of Toronto Press.

Friedman, M. and Friedman, R. (1980) *Free to Choose*, Harmondsworth: Penguin.

Friedmann, R. *et al.* (eds) (1987) *Modern Welfare States*, London: Harvester-Wheatsheaf.

Fukuyama, F. (1989) 'The end of history?' *The National Interest*, 16, Summer.

Galbraith, J.K. (1967) *The New Industrial State*, Harmondsworth: Penguin.

Gelb, J. (1990) 'Feminism and political action' in R.J. Dalton and M. Kuechler (eds) *Challenging the Political Order*, New York: Oxford University Press.

George, V. and Wilding, P. (1976) *Ideology and Social Welfare*, London: Routledge.

Gilder, G. (1982) *Wealth and Poverty*, New York: Bantam Books.

Gough, I. (1979) *The Political Economy of the Welfare State*, London: Macmillan.

Habermas, J. (1976) *Legitimation Crisis*, London: Heinemann.

—— (1981) 'New social movements', *Telos* 49.

Heclo, H. (1981) 'Toward a new welfare state?' in P. Flora and A.J. Heidenheimer (eds) *The Development of Welfare States in Europe and America*, New Brunswick: Transaction Books.

Heclo, H. and Madsden, H. (1987) *Policy and Politics in Sweden*, Philadelphia: Temple University Press.

Keane, J. and Owens, J. (1986) *After Full Employment*, London: Hutchinson.

Kerr, C. *et al.* (1960) *Industrialism and Industrial Man*, Cambridge, Mass.: Harvard University Press.

King, D.S. (1987) *The New Right*, London: Macmillan.

Korpi, W. (1978) *The Working Class in Welfare Capitalism*, London: Routledge.

—— (1983) *The Democratic Class Struggle*, London: Routledge.

Kuttner, R. (1984) *The Economic Illusion*, Boston: Houghton, Mifflin.

Lash, C. and Urry, J. (1987) *The End of Organised Capitalism*, Madison: University of Wisconsin Press.

Legrand, J. and Winter, D. (1987) 'The middle classes and the defence of the British welfare state' in R.E. Goodin and J. Legrand, *et al.*, *Not Only the Poor*, London: Allen & Unwin.

Lehmbruch, G. (1982) 'Introduction: neo-corporatism in comparative perspective' in G. Lehmbruch and P.C. Schmitter (eds) *Patterns of Corporatist Policy-Making*, London and Beverly Hills: Sage.

Lipset, S.M. (1960) *Political Man*, London: Heinemann.
Lyotard, J.F. (1984) *The Postmodern Condition: A Report on Knowledge*, Minneapolis: University of Minnesota Press.
Martin, A. (1986) 'The politics of employment and welfare' in K.G. Banting (ed.) *The State and Economic Interests*, Toronto: University of Toronto Press.
Milne, D. (1990) 'Canada's constitutional odyssey' in M.S. Whittington and G. Williams (eds) *Canadian Politics in the 1990s*, Scarborough: Nelson Canada.
Mishra, R. (1981) *Society and Social Policy*, London: Macmillan.
—— (1984) *The Welfare State in Crisis*, Brighton: Wheatsheaf Books.
—— (1990) *The Welfare State in Capitalist Society*, London: Harvester-Wheatsheaf.
Moody, K. (1987) 'Reagan, the business agenda and the collapse of labour' in R. Miliband *et al.* (eds) *Socialist Register 1987*, London: Merlin Press.
O'Connor, J. (1973) *The Fiscal Crisis of the State*, New York: St Martin's Press.
Offe, C. (1984) (ed. J. Keane) *Contradictions of the Welfare State*, Cambridge, Mass.: MIT Press.
—— (1985) 'New social movements', *Social Research* 52(4).
Olofsson, G. (1988) 'After the working-class movement?' *Acta Sociologica* 31(1).
Olsson, S.E. (1990) *Social Policy and Welfare State in Sweden*, Lund: Arkiv.
Organisation for Economic Co-operation and Development (1990) *Economic Outlook*, No. 48, December, Paris: OECD
—— (1991) *Economic Outlook: Historical Statistics* 1960–1989, Paris: OECD
Panitch, L. (1986) 'The tripartite experience' in K.G. Banting (ed.) *The State and Economic Interests*, Toronto: University of Toronto Press.
Panitch, L. and Swartz, D. (1985) *From Consent to Coercion*, Toronto: Garamond Press.
Pierson, C. (1990) 'The "exceptional" United States: first new nation or last welfare state', *Social Policy and Administration* 24(3).
Piven, F.F. and Cloward, R.A. (1985) *The New Class War*, New York: Pantheon Books.
Pontusson, J. (1984) 'Behind and beyond social democracy in Sweden', *New Left Review* 143.
—— (1987) 'Radicalization and retreat in Swedish social democracy', *New Left Review* 165.
Pratt, H.J. (1983) 'National interest groups among the elderly' in W.P. Browne and L.K. Olson (eds) *Aging and Public Policy*, Westport, Conn.: Greenwood Press.
Room, G. (1979) *The Sociology of Welfare*, Oxford: Blackwell.
Rucht, D. (1990) 'The strategies and action repertoires of new movements' in R.J. Dalton and M. Kuechler (eds) *Challenging the Political Order*, New York: Oxford University Press.
Salisbury, R.H. (1979) 'Why not corporations in America?' in P.C. Schmitter and G. Lehmbruch (eds) *Trends Towards Corporatist Intermediation*, London and Beverly Hills: Sage.
Schmitter, P.C. (1989) 'Corporatism is dead! Long live corporatism', *Government and Opposition* 24(1).
Simonsen, K. (1990) 'Planning on "postmodern conditions" ', *Acta Sociologica* 33(1).
Sombart, W.A. (1976) *Why Is There No Socialism in the United States?* New York: M.E. Sharpe.
Steinfels, P. (1979) *The Neoconservatives*, New York: Simon & Schuster.
Stephens, J.D. (1979) *The Transition from Capitalism to Socialism*, London: Macmillan.

Therborn, G. (1984) 'The prospects of labour and the transformation of advanced capitalism', *New Left Review* 145.

—— (1986) *Why Some Peoples Are More Unemployed Than Others*, London: Verso.

Therborn, G. and Roebroek, J. (1986) 'The irreversible welfare state', *International Journal of Health Services* 16 (3).

Thornburn, H.C. (1985) 'Interpretations of the Canadian party system' and 'Appendix' in H.C. Thornburn (ed.) *Party Politics in Canada*, Scarborough: Prentice-Hall Canada.

Walters, P. (1985) 'Distributing decline', *Government and Opposition* 20(3).

Weir, M., Orloff, A.S. and Skocpol, T. (1988) 'Introduction: understanding American social politics' in M. Weir, A.S. Orloff and T. Skocpol (eds) *The Politics of Social Policy in the United States*, Princeton, NJ: Princeton University Press.

Wilson, G.K. (1982) 'Why is there no corporatism in the United States?' in G. Lehmbruch and P.C. Schmitter (eds) *Patterns of Corporatist Policy-Making*, London and Beverly Hills: Sage.

Part II
Issues from Britain

3   Developments in social security policy

Jonathan Bradshaw

INTRODUCTION

Comparative social security research is still in its infancy. Considering the proportion of national revenues of the industrialised countries devoted to social security, the importance of social security to the living standards of their populations, and the acknowledged problems of administering social security expenditures in efficient and effective ways, it is extraordinary how little comparative research in the field is mounted. One of the consequences of this is that it is well nigh impossible to analyse how social security policy and its effects in the UK compare with other countries in Europe. Nevertheless this chapter contains a review of the comparative evidence that exists concerning the outcomes of social security policy.

TRENDS IN SOCIAL SECURITY IN THE UK

During the 1980s social security policy was in the hands of a government committed to so-called New Right ideologies. As King (1987) has pointed out, the New Right in Britain possesses not one single ideology but a collection of economic, political, moral and social beliefs that combine economic liberalism with a conservative commitment to traditional structures. Given the diversity of the ideas it is not surprising that it is not easy to explicate a coherent set of objectives for social security policy. Nevertheless it is possible to identify some aspirations that have had relevance to social security (Bradshaw, 1992). First it has been a fundamental tenet of New Right thinking that public expenditure at the beginning of the decade was too high, crowding out private consumption and investment, undermining personal incentives and harming the economy. There was also a view that the welfare state was wasteful and dominated by a self-serving bureaucracy and that help should be concentrated where it was needed most. These beliefs might be expected to have led to a number of policy measures in the field of social security – real reductions in expenditure, cuts in the level of benefits, an increase in selectivity, a concentration on improving work incentives and an extension of privatisation. All these objectives have been pursued with varying degrees of success.

However, what changes the government aspired to make in social security policy had to be made in the context of substantial constraints. These have included the demographic pressures from increasing numbers of pensioners, lone parents and people claiming disability benefits. Perhaps more important has been the unprecedented level of unemployment throughout the decade. The government has also been constrained politically by the very substantial level of public support that exists for public services (Jowell, *et al*., 1991).

What in the face of these constraints did the government achieve in the field of social security?

Social security expenditure has grown in cash terms, in real terms and as a proportion of GDP. Considerable efforts were made to reduce expenditure. After 1980 benefits were uprated by prices rather than earnings, some benefits were not uprated regularly, some benefits were abolished, others were phased out and entitlement to certain benefits was withdrawn for certain claimants. Social security expenditure continued to increase, however, partly owing to unemployment, partly owing to increased dependency of other groups, but also because of policy changes the government itself introduced.

There is no doubt that the social security policies pursued by the government have, in the context of high levels of unemployment, borne very hard on a large number of people, including, in particular, young people, students, the unemployed and families with children. The gap between the living standards of social security claimants and those in work has widened, the number of people living on low incomes has increased and, depending on the poverty threshold used, there has been a sharp increase in the number of people in relative poverty and no evidence that absolute poverty has diminished. There is also evidence that long-term post-war trends towards the greater equality of incomes was reversed after 1979 and the share of income of the top quintile group has increased at the expense of the bottom two quintile groups (Central Statistical Office, 1991).

The Conservative aspiration to concentrate help where it is needed most has been pursued through the expansion of the role of means-tested benefits – Income Support, Family Credit and Housing Benefit. However, most of the increase in dependency on means-tested benefits was the result of economic conditions and demographic changes. In a European context the British social security system has always been more reliant on income testing and it has become more and more reliant on means tests since the war (Deacon and Bradshaw, 1983). Despite the Conservative Government's commitment to selectivity, the bulk of the non-means-tested social security system remains intact for pensioners and the unemployed – and if anything it has been extended for the disabled. Although there have been many attempts to improve work incentives for those on benefit by cuts in benefits to the unemployed, tougher employment controls and improvements in benefits for those in low-paid work, the Conservative commitment to selectivity has led to a huge increase in the numbers of families with very high marginal tax rates as a result of the interaction of the tax/benefit system.

Privatisation has been pursued in a number of ways. Thus there has been a transfer of responsibility from the state to parents for the support of young people and students. More families have had to cover more of their own needs as the extra help to claimants of social assistance has been replaced by loans. Responsibility for paying benefits, but not financing them, has been transferred to employers. The most important element of privatisation, however has been in the provision of retirement pensions. Massive tax incentives have been used to encourage people to opt out of the State Earnings Related Pension Scheme into personal pension schemes. However, the government stepped back from an attempt to abolish the State Earnings Related Pensions Scheme and there is reason to expect that there will be a good deal of drifting back into the state scheme over time.

So, despite their aspirations and the rhetoric, social security has remained fairly impervious to the most radical government in Britain since the war. Since 1979 the structure of social security has changed but at the end of the day it is not so very different from before. The contributory and earnings-related elements may have become less important and therefore the system may have become less 'European'. But there is still a substantial insurance element in British social security as well as some interesting developments in non-contributory entitlements. The results of tax and benefit changes may have made Britain a less solidaristic nation, less equal, with more poverty. But the safety net is still there and probably more secure than in many other countries in Europe. Young people under 18 have been excluded, but in many European countries young people under 18 have never been covered anyway by social security.

Social security in Britain has certainly not become as residual and ineffective as the system in the USA. Indeed, it has proved itself an extraordinarily robust institution, firmly embedded in the social and cultural life of the country. If this conclusion is correct, then it must have implications for the chances of it changing radically in the face of the aspirations of the European Community to incorporate social security policies. This will be discussed further below, but meanwhile what challenges are facing social security in the UK over the next ten years?

THE FUTURE OF SOCIAL SECURITY IN BRITAIN

It is certainly the case that the main short-term variable governing the future of social security in Britain is the political persuasion of the government in power. Had the Labour Party regained power, there would have been firm commitments to increase pensions and Child Benefit and to restore the link between benefits and earnings. A new scheme for disability would have been introduced and no doubt the Social Fund would have been abolished, the future of the State Earnings Related Pension Scheme (SERPS) assured and earnings-related unemployment benefit reintroduced. There were also changes proposed for Housing Benefit, Income Support and benefits for those over 75. Labour also intended to divorce rights to some existing social insurance benefits from the contributory principle.

With Conservatives returned it is difficult to tell at this stage what new measures they might introduce. They are already committed to a new system of benefits for the disabled and a new agency to collect maintenance from absent parents. With Mrs Thatcher gone and a more One Nation feel about the government, it looks as if they might pursue rather more pragmatic policies with an emphasis on service to the customer.

Irrespective of party, government will have to face up to inevitable increases in expenditure arising from demographic changes, which will be mainly in the direction of an increasing proportion of elderly in the population (Bradshaw, 1991). In addition, of crucial importance, is what will happen to unemployment. This will depend on economic policy, national and international trends and changes in labour demand. But social security policy will also have to adapt to the changes that have been taking place in the labour market – a shift of emphasis from male, permanent, full-time jobs in manufacturing to female, part-time, temporary jobs in the service sector. The social security system has begun to adapt to these trends with the development of supplements to low earnings, but there is highly likely to be need for action on child care and on training and retraining, particularly if the labour market loosens again at the end of the present recession.

Pressure is also likely to build up for the equalisation of pension ages, and indeed the government has already expressed a commitment to the basic principle. However, the political and/or economic costs of any changes are likely to be considerable. There is likely to be a steady improvement in the operation of social security as the new Agencies (bodies somewhat detached from the central civil service and with a primary responsibility to serve the customer) become established and information technology is extended throughout the system.

But the major question-mark about the future development of social security – and the one of most relevance here – concerns what impact

European institutions will have on social security policy. During the 1980s these influences have tended to emanate from the European Court of Justice, whose decisions have led to increases in expenditure on benefits for the disabled through the imposition of 'equal treatment'. The impact of the Barber decision, which ruled that pensionable ages of men and women should be equalised, could be even more dramatic, although, in the short term, its impact is on the private sector. So the European Court could have a substantial impact particularly on the UK social security system, so much of which is governed by law and published regulation rather than administrative codes, as for instance in France.

THE IMPACT OF THE EUROPEAN COMMUNITY (EC)

Until recently, social security policy had never been a particularly salient aspect of the EC. True, the Treaty of Paris in 1951 had a commitment to improving working and living conditions. Also the Treaty of Rome mentioned the harmonisation of social security. In practice, however, the interest of the EC in social policy issues was restricted almost exclusively to measures concerned with the labour market, in particular the movement of labour and its social security implications. Far from harmonisation, the aspiration has merely been to limit divergence.

Part of the explanation for this lies in the origins of the EC, which were largely concerned with economic cooperation. It is also partly explained by conflicts in the institutional framework, with, in particular, the Council of Ministers striving to rein back the Commission in the context of a largely ineffective European Parliament. It is also the case that social security policy varies considerably throughout the EC and is an intimate product of national experience, history, culture and traditions. Because of the popularity of national programmes, governments are likely to remain reluctant to permit a shift in the balance of authority too far towards supranational institutions.

However, a number of factors have led to change. The experience of the 'Crisis in the Welfare State' in all countries led to an increased realisation that the countries of the EC had common problems that called for shared solutions. With the extension of the Community came an increased awareness that living standards varied substantially and that social security policy played a vital part in the distribution of resources geographically. Also there was anxiety that the richer countries might be the victims of social dumping by the poorer countries or their peoples. The EC has begun to recognise that the population of Europe consists not merely of workers but also of productive and less productive people outside the paid workforce such as children, those rearing children and the retired. The European Parliament has been slowly growing in confidence. The idea that the

Community should stand for higher aspirations than merely better living standards through economic growth has been catching on. The rights of women, the needs of the disabled and the treatment of the unemployed have become foci of concern. Increasingly it was recognised that the EC was boring, that it was failing to catch the imagination of people – and that it needed to develop a human face if it was going to survive. The European Court of Justice, ahead of other institutions of the Community, was being used to advance social rights through test cases. It adopted this role with liberal interpretation and vigorous enforcement and has been prepared to contemplate individuals bringing suits on a wide range of alleged violations of the Treaty.

But the movement to implement these new aspirations has been extremely tentative, if not lethargic. However, after almost two decades it eventually resulted in the Single European Act in 1987. This Act, which is due to come into effect at the end of 1992, signals an advance in social and economic cohesion and the introduction of a European Social Dimension. The discussion surrounding these measures has still been very preoccupied with employment and regional policy, but there has been a growing concern over vulnerable communities, groups and regions, a desire that the poor of Europe should not be excluded and a recognition that social security policy had a role to play in all of this.

The British government has throughout been a fairly reluctant partner. Most attention has been given in the media to the government's anxieties about the Fundamental Charter for Social Rights, the Exchange Rate Mechanism and the Single European Currency. But the British government has also been fighting a less well-publicised rearguard action over the attempts of the Commission to obtain acceptance of directives affecting specific social security policies. There have been numerous examples, including an attempt during the Greek Presidency in 1990, to impose a directive that all workers, however low their earnings, should be included in national insurance schemes; also an attempt, during the Dutch Presidency in 1991, to advance rights to maternity leave. The British are signatories of the Single European Act, but they are opposed to many of the attempts by other countries to implement it – on two main grounds.

The first is really highly ideological and stems from an anxiety that part of the EC agenda is to reassert the power of labour, which the Conservative government has taken such pains to undermine. Extending the rights of workers would, it has been argued by the British government, stifle enterprise and lose British jobs. The government has been anxious to encourage labour market flexibility and deregulation and to *avoid* much more intervention.

The second objection stems from a mixture of constitutional anxieties and nationalism – a belief that social policies are most appropriately reserved to national governments, being part of the machinery of politics, not something to be imposed on free nations and their parliaments by supranational bodies. Here the British government seeks to invoke the catholic (and therefore to an extent alien) doctrine of subsidiarity. This doctrine, as it relates to the EC, is that decisions should not be taken at any higher level than they need to be. Or rather that the UK Parliament should be left alone to determine its own social security policy. As Spicker (1991:12) points out:

> there is some inconsistency in arguing that the EC can intervene supranationally in economic affairs but could not have a case for intervening supranationally in social affairs and one has to be suspicious of a principle which seems to limit the actions of the EC and almost no one else .

There is probably something to be learned in this from the development of federal systems elsewhere, notably in the US and Canada. Subsidiarity may have been a starting principle in each case, yet eventually the centre has taken increasing power in order to control and limit variation, using its greater resources as 'bribes' to this effect.

COMPARATIVE RESEARCH IN SOCIAL SECURITY

It is probable that one of the explanations for the so far tentative involvement of the EC in social security policy, and also the difficulties inherent in predicting the future role that the EC might play, is the lack of good comparative data on social security in Europe.

There are two sources of funding for comparative research: national governments and international organisations.

National governments

In order to sustain reciprocal agreements, governments need to know about the social security arrangements in other countries. However, the depth of the knowledge that they need does not call for research as such, merely a knowledge of entitlements at an individual level. Governments may also want to have some view about how they compare in the resources devoted to social security with other countries – particularly because of the importance of social security in the distribution of gross domestic product (see below).

National governments may want to launch comparative studies of social security – in order to 'learn from abroad'. But such studies in Britain during the 1980s have been few and far between. The Conservative government has not been much interested in domestic social security research – let alone in how Britain compares with other countries. All the same there have been flurries of interest in what is being done elsewhere. For example Mr Fowler visited France in order to learn from the arrangements there for the unemployed. (At the time France did not give benefits to unemployed people who did not have a contribution record.) Similarly visits were made to the USA to study Workfare, and the Child Support Act was informed by the arrangements existing in Australia and Wisconsin to ensure that absent parents pay some maintenance to former partners and children.

The curiosity of the British government may now be increasing. The departure of the spirit of Thatcherism, with its particular nationalism, has led to a more open sense of enquiry and this may well be having an impact. Certainly there is evidence that the Department of Social Security (DSS) is beginning to take more of an interest in arrangements overseas and to show a willingness to contemplate comparative studies – not least now that 1992 is upon us.

International organisations

In the absence of a contribution from national governments to comparative research in social security we have to turn to the international organisations. The Organisation for Economic Co-Operation and Development (OECD) undertakes a variety of comparative research for its members and without doubt it has made considerable effort in the 1980s to assess the impact of social expenditure on industrialised economies. However, the OECD is dominated by economists and an international macro agenda where, perhaps unwisely, social security is perceived as a marginal player. Most of the OECD's analysis is certainly at a macro level, concerned with inputs: the level of taxes and benefits paid by the average earner, the proportion of GDP devoted to social transfers, the consequences of demographic change for social expenditure (OECD, 1985, 1988a, 1988b, 1988c, 1990). Only fairly recently has it begun to focus on micro issues and on the outcomes of social expenditure for particular client groups. Thus a collection of essays has been published by the OECD on the treatment of lone parents (Duskin, 1990) and a new project is in train to assess the impact of growing dependency on social security policy.

The International Social Security Association (ISSA) provides an official forum, a research review and a journal and produces a compendium of social security arrangements around the world, which is, curiously, published by the US federal government.

The European Community – for all that it has been committed to harmonising social arrangements since the early 1950s – undertakes remarkably little comparative research in social security. Eurostat, the statistical office, is increasingly producing relevant data, particularly on poverty. Some specific studies focusing on social security policy have been funded by the EC (Bradshaw and Piachaud, 1980; Roll, 1990), but most of the effort and resources in the EC poverty programmes have gone into local community action projects. Some people believe that this has been a major error, enabling the structural causes of poverty to be overlooked and the real differences in national governments' treatment of the poor to be hidden. Thereby the Community has failed to further the interests of the poor with quality comparative research on living standards, income distribution and social security.

For some years the EC has produced its *Social Protection in the Member States of the Community* (EEC/MISSOC, 1991). But this has been of very limited analytical value because the editions have taken so long to emerge. There are signs, however, that the attitude of the EC to comparative research is changing. The Commission, in its Action Programme relating to the implementation of the Community Charter of Fundamental Social Rights for Workers, is stressing the need for convergence in social security schemes. The Commission has decided that an essential prerequisite for such a convergence process is reliable and up-to-date information. It is now committed to producing the comparative tables more rapidly and a group of officials from the member states act as informants to update these every year. This means that they can and have been used in a limited way to examine differences in levels of benefits between member states (Roll, 1991).

DESCRIPTIVE SOCIAL SECURITY RESEARCH

Most of the best comparative academic research on social security has been descriptive; at least descriptive of social security systems, with relatively little attention paid to their outcomes. Gordon's (1988) work is a remarkable achievement. She draws on the compendium published by the US Department of Health and Human Services for ISSA in 1985. Unfortunately much of this material is old. For example, the UK data are for 1982 and mainly relate to the early 1980s if not earlier still. The second half of the 1980s has seen changes in social security in many countries, including unprecedented levels of unemployment, the growing burden of ageing, radical changes in the pattern of family life and, in many countries, new kinds of policy pursued by New Right regimes. The abiding problem with descriptive studies of social security is that they are not really designed to be historical – rather they seek to compare and contrast what exists now. So if 'now' is too far away, these comparisons are of correspondingly limited value in a rapidly changing time.

To overcome the problems faced by Gordon, descriptive comparative social security needs to be tackled on a narrower basis: either a few countries or a few policies or both. A number of studies have focused on a particular type of social security and tackled it from a comparative perspective. There are for example the series of studies by Kamerman and Kahn, who over the years, have taken a limited number of countries and specific policy areas – such as family policy – and, with the help of national experts, undertaken detailed comparisons (see, for example, Kamerman and Kahn, 1983; Kahn and Kamerman, 1983). There are similar studies of pensions (Wilson, 1974), benefits for the unemployed (Mitton and Lawson, 1983), child support (Bradshaw and Piachaud, 1980), and benefits for lone-parent families (Millar, 1989) and for working-age women (Millar, 1991). These studies vary as to the number of countries covered and in the methods they employ. However, there is an increasing tendency to employ national informants working to a predetermined analytical structure and to use model families to ensure that like is being compared with like. Even so, there are a number of problems with such studies.

First, they are invariably launched as one-off exercises and not updated over time. They therefore soon get out of date. Furthermore, none of the compendia have been able to proceed from the description of benefit systems to an analysis of their value for model families. The sole exception to this is the OECD, which produces a regular analysis of the impact of taxes and family benefits on a number of model families at national average income (OECD, 1990) that can be used to assess their impact on model families.

Second, these descriptive studies tend to give the formal or official position rather than a portrayal of what happens in practice. Thus, for example, they assume that where a benefit exists it is taken up. Again, the use of model families inevitably involves a host of assumptions about, for example, the number and ages of children, whether the adults work, their wage rates and hours, their housing tenure and costs. The accumulation of such assumptions makes it most unlikely that the model family actually exists in practice. Nevertheless these types of descriptive studies are of enormous help in advancing the understanding of benefit systems in different countries and their impact on families and individuals. They also enable us to understand how packages of benefits interact and how social security interacts both with the wage system and with systems of taxation and tax allowances. The better studies of this type also take into account the value of housing subsidies and services in kind.

SOCIAL SECURITY RESEARCH RELATED TO OUTCOMES

A variety of comparative schools have sought to establish the outcomes of social security policy.

First, there are those who have been concerned with the comparative analysis of welfare states. The focus of their work has not been restricted to social security. The effort has progressed from the analysis of public expenditure as a proportion of domestic product to the analysis of the structure of social security expenditure. These types of comparison have been influential in demonstrating that the UK does not have a particularly high proportion of GDP devoted to public expenditure, that social expenditure as a proportion of public expenditure is comparatively low, that expenditure on transfers as opposed to expenditure on goods and services is very low, that a larger proportion of transfers are means tested rather than contributory, that a larger proportion of benefit expenditure is funded from direct and particularly indirect tax as opposed to contributions and that the UK faces a relatively more manageable demographic outlook over the next 40 or 50 years than many other countries (see, for example, Cameron, 1985; Gilbert and Moon, 1988; Heidenheimer *et al.,* 1990; Flora, 1986; Dixon and Scheurall, 1989; Ringen, 1987). This type of research has been an important source of evidence to counter the aspirations of politicians informed by New Right ideology to blame government overload, the level of social expenditure and high rates of taxation for the poor performance of their economies. However, this research inevitably has its limits. The data are invariably out of date by the time of publication. Most of these data are derived from national accounts, so there are horrendous problems in ensuring that like is being compared with like. Most important of all it has become clear that to understand the effectiveness of social security policy, its outputs and outcomes, and to form a view of the efficiency and effectiveness of different systems in achieving their objectives, calls for an analysis of micro social data.

There are those who have used micro social data to explore the impact of social security. The essence of this work is that data derived from surveys of the income and/or expenditure of individuals, households and families at national level are used to compare countries. Probably the most common application of this type of research has been to compare poverty rates in different countries – for all that the reduction of poverty is not everywhere by any means a declared policy objective.

The European Commission financed three studies in 1976, 1983 and 1989 on perceptions of poverty. Overall the proportion of the population in the EC perceiving themselves to be poor increased from 7.6 per cent in 1976 to 10.7 per cent in 1983 and then fell back again to 8.6 per cent in 1989 (Figure 3.1).

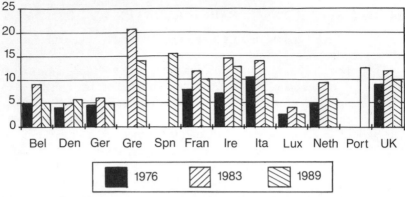

Figure 3.1 Percentage of households perceiving themselves as poor or near poor, 1976, 1983 and 1989
Source: European Commission.

The figures for the UK were 9.3, 11.5 and 9.8 per cent respectively (EC 1991). In 1989 the proportion feeling themselves poor in the UK was similar to that in France, but much larger than the proportions in Italy, the Netherlands, Luxembourg, West Germany, Denmark and Belgium.

The EC, as part of its Programmes to Combat Poverty, commissioned an analysis of the numbers of people and proportions of each population living in poverty. Respondents in each country were asked to re-analyse their own data sets using common definitions of the unit of analysis, income, expenditure and so on, and then to count the number falling below a common poverty level, which was set at the proportion of the population living below 50 per cent of the median income. Estimates using an income definition have been produced for 1975, 1980 and 1985 (O'Higgins and Jenkins, 1989). Whereas in the *Final Report on the Second European Poverty Programme 1985–1989* (EC, 1991) estimates are produced on the basis of an expenditure and an income threshold, Figure 3.2 shows the incidence of child poverty as measured by the numbers of children living in families with total equivalent expenditure of less than 50 per cent of the average. The UK comes third after Portugal and Ireland in the proportion of children below this standard in 1985, and, after the Netherlands, shows the sharpest increase between 1980 and 1985.

Figure 3.3 uses the average Community definition (equivalent expenditure) as the poverty line and now the UK performs rather better. But it still has a considerably larger proportion of children living in poverty than all the 'northern' EC countries including Italy.

The results obtained from these comparative studies of poverty depend on the indicator of living standards employed, the threshold taken as the poverty

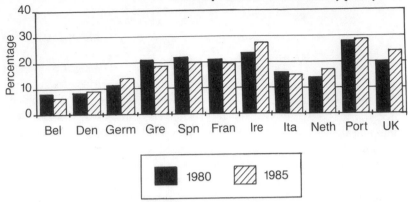

Figure 3.2 Incidence of poverty among children, 1980 and 1985. Poverty line equal to 50% of national average equivalent expenditure
Source: European Commission (1991).

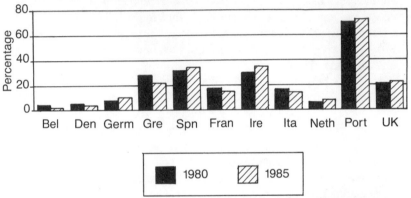

Figure 3.3 Incidence of poverty among children, 1980 and 1985. Poverty line equal to 50% of the Community average equivalent expenditure at 1980
Source: European Commission (1991).

line, the choice of unit of analysis, the choice of equivalence scale and, in particular, whether the focus is on poverty numbers (the number living below a threshold) or poverty gaps (the distance between their income and the threshold). Over and above these quasi technical, even arcane, issues, as Atkinson (1991) has pointed out, poverty-line studies really need to be complemented by studies of how people actually live in different countries. Deleek and colleagues (1991) have been evaluating four different poverty lines based on original micro studies in seven EC countries, while Hagenaas and de Vos (1988) have demonstrated that it is possible to obtain quite different results using different definitions of poverty.

There is still a good way to go in producing fully comparable data sets appropriate for the analysis of poverty. However, the use of such comparative data sets is expanding. Rainwater, Rein and Schwartz (1986) used micro data from several countries. Their book used data tapes from the US Panel Study of Income Dynamics for 1971, the UK General Household Survey for 1973 and the Swedish Level of Living Survey for 1968 to compare how the incomes of families in the three countries are made up and *inter alia* the contribution of social security. Their study was a precursor to the much more substantial comparative project based on the accumulated micro data sets in the Luxembourg Income Study (LIS). At Luxembourg a coalition of researchers led by Smeeding and Rainwater has established comparable data sets for, now, 16 countries. Two instalments of the data are so far available. Analysis based on the first, covering data around 1980, has now begun to reach publication (see, for example, Smeeding, O'Higgins and Rainwater, 1990; Mitchell, 1991; Smeeding *et al.*, 1989). The second instalment of data, relating to *c.* 1985, is now available for analysis. With the passage of time the data sets are becoming more fully comparable and researchers using them can be increasingly confident that the 60 or so income and demographic variables included have been drawn from national surveys using a common framework.

One of the best analyses of this kind of data is that of Mitchell. She has published an analysis of the 1980 material (Mitchell, 1991) and Mitchell and Bradshaw (1992) have employed the 1985 data to examine the outcomes of tax/benefit policy in reducing poverty and inequality amongst lone parents. This work demonstrates that the LIS data enable the impact of both social security transfers and income taxes to be assessed together and separately. It is also possible to assess the contribution of alternative instruments: for example to compare means-tested and universal benefits, or child benefits and child tax allowances. It is also possible to assess the efficiency with which redistribution is achieved: how well transfers are targeted, for instance, and how much redistribution is achieved for each pound spent on social security.

Evaluation of the extent to which poverty is reduced (Table 3.1) depends to some extent on the poverty line used – whether it is 40, 50 or 60 per cent of median income. Taking the 50 per cent poverty measure, the UK comes eighth (out of 10) in pre-transfer poverty rank and fourth in post-transfer poverty rates. If the 40 per cent line is taken, however, the UK comes third lowest in the proportion of families below post-transfer poverty lines, whereas if the 60 per cent level is taken the UK comes fourth in the post-transfer poverty league table.

Compared with the other LIS countries the UK has a low proportion of the poor (taking poverty as below 50 per cent of the median income) who are aged and single and a much higher proportion of couples with children (Table 3.2).

Table 3.1 Percentage of families in poverty (below a proportion of median equivalent net income), pre-and post- transfer, *c.* 1985

Country	Below 40% median		Below 50% median		Below 60% median	
	Pre-transfer	Post-transfer	Pre-transfer	Post-transfer	Pre-transfer	Post-transfer
Australia	25.8	6.2	27.5	10.0	30.5	21.3
Canada	23.0	6.8	26.4	11.7	30.1	17.7
France	33.9	5.1	39.1	8.3	44.4	13.8
Germany	33.5	2.6	35.3	6.3	36.8	13.2
Italy	33.3	5.2	36.9	9.8	42.9	17.3
Luxembourg	31.2	1.9	35.5	5.4	41.3	11.3
Netherlands	31.2	4.6	32.3	5.9	34.0	9.6
Sweden	34.6	5.4	37.6	7.6	40.7	12.6
UK	35.5	4.1	37.3	6.9	39.7	12.8
USA	24.2	12.7	27.9	18.5	31.8	24.9

Source: Mitchell and Bradshaw (1992).

Table 3.2 Composition of the poor (below 50 per cent median equivalent net income) population by family type – *c.* 1985

Country	Aged single	Aged couple	Single	Couple	Lone parent	Couple+ children	Other	Total
Australia	5.0	5.2	20.0	12.0	20.4	35.4	2.0	100.0
Canada	3.8	2.8	33.8	9.9	16.2	28.4	5.0	100.0
France	1.3	1.7	20.4	23.9	7.1	40.7	4.9	100.0
Germany	11.8	10.2	21.6	17.4	7.9	26.2	4.9	100.0
Italy	6.1	6.3	2.9	25.0	2.6	47.9	9.2	100.0
Luxembourg	13.5	17.6	9.7	19.2	6.4	33.1	0.5	100.0
Netherlands	0.0	0.4	49.0	9.4	4.9	33.3	3.1	100.0
Sweden	5.7	1.7	80.8	4.3	1.3	6.2	–	100.0
UK	1.4	2.8	9.9	19.0	8.9	53.4	4.5	100.0
USA	13.6	5.0	21.0	8.5	21.9	24.2	5.8	100.0

Source: Mitchell and Bradshaw (1992).

The poverty rate – the proportion of the population living below a given line – is a head count measure. Yet as important in comparing a country's performance in poverty alleviation, is the extent to which the transfer system closes the poverty gap. In the mid-1980's the UK has the third largest post-transfer poverty gap as a proportion of GDP of all the countries in the study (Table 3.3).

Next, Table 3.4 compares the success of the LIS countries in reducing inequalities as measured by Gini coefficients. Pre-transfer, the UK ranks with Sweden and France as the most unequal *c.* 1985. After the impact of social security transfers, the UK is less unequal than the USA, France and

Mitchell's work also illustrates the limitations of LIS. Once again, like most comparative data on social security, it is out of date. However, now most of the bugs in the operation have been sorted out, one can expect subsequent instalments of data to be available and produced more quickly. Even so, there are still some irreconcilable differences in respect of the way the data have been collected in different countries which limit the range of comparisons possible. Also, the data for different countries come in at slightly different stages of the business cycle, which again can mean that like is not being compared with like.

To date, comparative analysis of micro data has not been able to take into account the value of services in kind in the way that the CSO analysis of the impact of taxes and benefits published in *Economic Trends*, for instance, estimates the value and distributional consequences of public expenditure (including tax expenditure) on housing, health and education. Work is in progress to deal with this defect in the LIS data. The results may make a good deal of difference to the ranking of the UK, since, as Whiteford (1991) has pointed out, the benefit of the NHS raised the equivalent disposable income of the lowest quintile of British households by 28 per cent in 1987 (CSO, 1991); and, at around the same time, British households were spending about 1.3 per cent of their average total expenditure on medical care and health expenses, compared with 6 per cent in Italy, 9 per cent in France, 11 per cent in Belgium, 13 per cent in the Netherlands and 15 per cent in West Germany. If such expenditures were taken into account, the relative ranking of UK families might indeed change.

The results obtained also raise questions about how and why such differences occur. The real challenge for comparative studies of social security is to be able to link the results obtained from the analysis of micro data with the kind of detailed understanding of the operation and interaction of taxes and benefits that comes from the descriptive studies discussed earlier.

CONCLUSION

What is going to happen to social security systems in the next couple of decades? The impact of economic and political reform in the Soviet Union and the countries of Eastern Europe will change the focus of the European Community profoundly. The process of integration and the possible movement of large bodies of workers from East to West will without doubt have an influence on the social policies and social security policies of the European Community. But what will be the influence of the rest of Europe on the UK? At present social policy remains one key area of policy left in the hands of the nation states. However, after decades of 'neglect', social policy and social security policy are now beginning to creep onto the supranational agenda and have the potential for being at the heart of the policies of the European Community. Though it is not yet clear that they will be.

Leibfried and Pierson (1992) have argued that there are now quite clear tendencies towards economic and political integration within the EC and that, if these continue, there must inevitably be pressures to develop something more than the present limited EC presence in social policy. Even so, there are good reasons to be sceptical about the potential of European institutions to bring about such change. They are fragmented and it is the opponents of reform who tend to occupy the political high ground. Furthermore, in many countries agencies – such as the trades unions – that might generate supranational change have themselves been diminished in the course of the 1980s. If they still have power to influence, it is an influence over what kind of policies hold sway rather than whether policies are developed at all. There is also the great heterogeneity of the EC to be considered – the enormous diversity of institutional goals, institutions and cultural aspirations. There is little uniformity within Europe as regards how money is spent or the purposes for which it is spent. If the EC is to enter at all into this great diversity, it will probably not be in the areas where policy has already been pre-empted by national governments – such as pensions, education and health care – but in areas where there is potential for change and where there is 'policy space' (such as in respect of policy for carers). The European Court of Justice may well be the vehicle through which unification is pioneered. It has extensive authority over its national counterparts and has already proved itself capable of radical decisions which, although they leave implementation in the hands of national governments, set the strategy of rights. So far, the EC has confined its attention on distributional issues to the well-being of selected groups – farmers through the CAP, populations in the poorer regions, the EC's own civil servants, and to some extent women (mainly through decisions of the European Court). There is a good deal of speculation about the importance of social protection, lots of conferences, some research but little action. If the activity of the Community continues to be driven by market considerations it is possible that the EC role in social policy might continue to focus merely on the mobile worker, but this is unlikely. For the market to work, for there to be a 'level playing field', more is required from social policy than merely a mobile workforce. However, a further effort in comparative research is called for if we are to be informed about how best to move forward.

REFERENCES

Allen, E. and Bradshaw, J.R. (1991) 'Child support in the EC', *Poverty*, No. 80. Winter, 16.

Atkinson, A.B. (1991) *Poverty, Statistics and Progress in Europe*, Discussion Paper WSP/60, London School of Economics.

Bradshaw, J. (1991) 'Social security expenditure in the 1990s', *Public Money and Management* 11, (4), 25–31.

—— (1992) 'Social security' in D. Marsh, and R.A.W. Rhodes, (eds) *Implementing Thatcherite Policies: Audit of an Era*, Milton Keynes: Open University Press.

Bradshaw, J. and Piachaud, D. (1980) *Child Support in the European Community*, London: Bedford Square Press.

Cameron, D. (1985) 'Public expenditure and economic performance in international perspective' in R. Klein and M. O'Higgins (eds) *The Future of Welfare*, Oxford: Basil Blackwell.

Castles, F. and Mitchell, D. (1992). 'Identifying welfare state regimes: the links between politics, instruments and outcomes', *Governance* 5(1), 1–26.

Central Statistical Office (1991) 'The effects of taxes and benefits on household income, 1988', *Economic Trends* (London: HMSO), 449, March, 107–149.

Deacon, A. and Bradshaw, J. (1983) *Reserved for the Poor: The Means Test in British Social Policy*, Oxford: Martin Robertson.

Deleek, H. (1991) *The Measurement of Poverty in Comparative Context: empirical evidence and methodological evaluation of four poverty lines in seven EC countries*, Nordwijk, Netherlands: Poverty Statistics in European Community.

Dixon, J. and Scheurell, P. (eds) (1989) *Social Welfare in the Developed Market Countries*, London: Routledge & Kegan Paul.

Duskin, E. (ed.) (1990) *Lone Parent Families: The economic challenge*, Paris: OECD.

European Commission (1991) *Final Report on the Second European Poverty Programme 1985–1989*, COM(91) 29, Brussels.

EEC/MISSOC (1991) *Social Protection in the Member States of the Community*, European Commission.

Esping-Andersen, G. (1990) *The Three Worlds of Welfare Capitalism*, Oxford: Polity Press.

Flora, P. (1986) *Growth to the Limits: the Western European welfare states since World War II*, Vols I and II, Berlin: de Gruyter.

Gilbert, N. and Moon, A. (1988) 'Analysing welfare effort: an appraisal of comparative methods', *Journal of Policy Analysis and Management* 7(2), 328–32.

Gordon, M. (1988) *Social Security Policies in Industrial Countries. A Comparative Analysis*, Cambridge: Cambridge University Press.

Hagenaas, A. and de Vos, K. (1988) 'Definition and measurement of poverty', *Journal of Human Resources* 23, (2), 211–21.

Heidenheimer, A., Heclo, H. and Adams, C. (eds) (1990) *Comparative Public Policy*, 3rd edn, New York: St Martin's Press.

Jowell, R., Witherspoon, S., Brook, L. and Taylor, B. (1991) *British Social Attitudes, the 7th Report*, Aldershot: Gower.

Kahn A.J. and Kamerman, S.B. (1983) *Income Transfers for Families with Children*, Philadelphia: Temple University Press.

Kamerman, S.B. and Kahn, A.J. (eds) (1983) *Essays on Income Transfers and Related Programes in Eight Countries*, New York: Columbia University.

King, D.S. (1987) *The New Right: Politics, Markets and Citizenship*, London: Macmillan.

Leibfried, S. and Pierson, P. (1992) *Emergent Supranational Social Policy: The EC's Social Dimension*, Cambridge Mass.: Harvard University, Center for European Studies (forthcoming).

Millar, J. (1989) *Poverty and the Lone-Parent Family*, Aldershot: Avebury/Gower.
—— (1991) *Socio-economic Situations of Solo Women in Europe*, Brussels: European Commission.
Mitton, R. and Lawson, R. (1983) *Unemployment, Poverty and Social Policy*, London: Bedford Square Press.
Mitchell, D. (1991) *Income Transfers in Ten welfare states*, Aldershot: Avebury/Gower.
Mitchell, D. and Bradshaw, J. (1992) *Lone Parents and their Incomes: a Comparative Study of Ten Countries*, University of York (forthcoming).
OECD (1985) *Social Expenditure 1960–1990 – Problems of Growth and Control*, Paris.
—— (1988a) *Aging Population: the social security implications*, Paris.
—— (1988b) *Reforming Public Pensions*, Paris.
—— (1988c) *The Future of Social Protection*, Paris.
—— (1990) *Health Care Systems in Transition: the search for efficiency*, Paris.
O'Higgins, M. and Jenkins, S.P. (1989) *Poverty in Europe – Estimates for 1975–1985*, Nordwijk, Netherlands: Poverty Statistics in EC.
Rainwater, L., Rein, M. and Schwartz, J. (1986) *Income Packaging in the welfare state: a comparative study of family income*, Oxford: Clarendon Press.
Ringen, S. (1987) *The Possibility of Politics*, Oxford: Oxford University Press.
Roll, J. (1990) *Lone Parent Families in the European Community*, London: Family Policy Studies Centre.
—— (1991) *Benefiting Europe's Children*, London: Family Policy Studies Centre.
Smeeding, T., O'Higgins, M. and Rainwater, L. (1990) *Poverty, Inequality and Income Distribution in Comparative Perspective*, London: Harvester/Wheatsheaf.
Smeeding, T., Torrey, B. and Palmer, J. (eds) (1989) *The Vulnerable*, Washington DC: The Urban Institute.
Spicker, P. (1991) 'The principle of subsidiarity and the social policy of the European Community', *Journal of European Social Policy* 1, (1), 3–15.
Whiteford, P. (1991) Social Policy Research Unit paper, University of York, unpublished.
Wilson, T. (ed.) (1974) *Pensions, Inflation and Growth*, London: Heinemann.

4 Encouraging home ownership
Trends and prospects

John Doling

INTRODUCTION

The dominant feature of British housing policy in the 1980s was the promotion of home ownership. In 1979, when Mrs Thatcher formed her first government, 54.7 per cent of households were home owners (Department of the Environment, 1991). Ten years later the proportion had risen to 66.6 per cent, placing Britain close to the top of the Western industrialised nations' league table of home ownership. Since, over the same period, the local authority sector decreased from 31.4 per cent to 23.3 per cent, the 1980s was a decade in which there was a significant shift from state to market provision. These developments cannot be adequately explained as the result either of unguided, market forces or of the unintended consequences of other policies. Rather, they occurred mainly because they were deliberately fostered and explicitly supported.

How typical was the British experience? Writing at the outset of the 1990s, it is clear that, in pursuing policies in the 1980s ostensibly aimed in the general direction of increasing private forms of housing provision, and in actually achieving higher rates of home ownership, Britain has not been alone. Although the policy goals have not always been so transparent, many Western countries have pursued privatisation policies during at least some of the last two decades. It is, of course, not necessarily the case that private forms of housing provision are equated only with home ownership, since this would ignore private rental tenures in particular. Nevertheless, in practice, many other countries have also experienced long-term growth of home ownership. One consequence is that home ownership is now the numerically largest form of housing provision in many of the welfare states of the Western industrialised world.

The growing domination of home ownership may seem to suggest a process of convergence in housing systems, but the developments have been far from linear and there are, in fact, wide variations between countries.

Indeed, in many respects, for example in the relative sizes of home ownership sectors, these variations are as great now as they were in the early post-war years. Moreover, the continuation of these differences between countries may be more significant than the general tendency for home ownership to have grown. In searching for explanations for these differences a more promising avenue than convergence or stages of growth theories appears to be found in national ideological preferences. That is, that home ownership has been fostered most in those countries in which the ideological preference has been most consistent with, and in some cases centred on, the private ownership of property. On this view, therefore, the growth in home ownership in Britain in the 1980s has been engendered by an underlying ideological predilection which found expression in the policies of the Conservative government.

However, even with the continuation of a Conservative government, this does not mean that the further growth of home ownership is assured. The direction of future developments is uncertain, partly because, whatever objectives, if any, have been fulfilled by past developments, they have frequently been accompanied by a range of problems, such as widespread financial distress amongst home owners. In Britain – and, as this paper will show, sometimes elsewhere – the ideological has seemingly been confronted by the economic. Although there may be ideological pressures for continued growth, the economic environment may not always be consistent with, may indeed act against, growth. In these circumstances it is possible that there will be changes in policy directions in the 1990s. Certainly, whatever the post-war experience, there is no universal law that home ownership will always increase in advanced capitalist societies.

This paper considers four aspects of the long-term growth, and continued variation in the relative sizes, of home-owning sectors. First, it maps out the main policy developments in Britain in the 1980s which have enhanced the opportunities, as well as reduced the alternative opportunities, to enter home ownership. Second, it explores aspects of the similarity, and dissimilarity, of British developments to housing developments in other industrialised countries. It argues that these similarities and dissimilarities are founded in different national ideological structures. Third, the paper provides evidence, also in comparative perspective, of some of the economic difficulties for some individuals of pursuing home ownership strategies. The paper concludes by speculating about the range of future directions for housing policies and the consequences these directions might have for home ownership.

POLICIES FOR HOME OWNERSHIP IN BRITAIN

One view of the relative numerical significance of different tenures in a country is that it reflects the state's 'tenure strategy' (Kemeny, 1981). In using this term Kemeny has in mind the arrangements – such as the nature of housing banks and tenure-specific subsidies – that governments have introduced and that affect the balance of advantage and disadvantage of each tenure. In some countries individual households, deciding how best to meet their housing needs, will perceive the balance weighted in favour of home ownership, and in others weighted in favour of one or more forms of renting. Tenure decisions, then, are not determined by, but made in the context of, a (state-) guided market. Although Kemeny uses the word 'strategy', he suggests that any guidance or structure will be the result not of a comprehensive set of policies, implemented at one time with the objective of specified tenure outcomes, but of ad hoc government decisions taken at different points in time and in the context of the specific conditions pertaining at those points. Thus there is a sense in which any structure might be thought to be the outcome of tactics rather than of strategy.

It might be convincing to argue that in the two decades before 1979 the development of a tenure strategy or structure by government in Britain was largely ad hoc: that the introduction of subsidies favourable to the extension of home ownership, for example, was not part of any long-term housing goal but rather the by-product of other goals. In post-1979 Britain, however, such an argument would seem less convincing. Until at least the middle years of the decade, housing policy established a comprehensive and largely consistent structure which had as its central objective the transfer of houses from the public to the private, home-owning, sector, and which is perhaps best expressed in the Prime Minister's own words: 'What I am desperately trying to do is to create one nation with everyone being a man of property' (quoted by Young, 1983). Although this has been clearly part of a wider agenda about the nature of society as a whole, and about the centrality of macro-economic objectives and appropriate policies, the extension of home ownership has arguably been seen as desirable in its own right.

Although by the end of the decade there has been some refocusing of objectives, the package of policies introduced within the first two years of office clearly demonstrated the government's determination 'to explore the limits to the growth of home ownership (Malpass, 1990: 1). It had three elements that radically shifted the balance of advantage for individual households in favour of home ownership: by decreasing the number of alternative (rental) opportunities; by reducing entry costs; and by increasing the availability of finance. The first part of the change came in 1979 with the revision of public expenditure targets, which proposed cuts in the housing programme – principally consisting of spending on council housing. These cuts were proportionately greater than those for any other programme. The continuation of state stringency in this area has meant a reduction in the number of new public sector houses constructed from almost 75,000 in 1979 to under 14,000 in 1989 (Department of the Environment, 1991). (There was also a reduction, though less severe, in construction by housing associations, which in Britain are part of the non-profit or social housing sector.) Alongside the reduction in new building which limited the new opportunities to enter this sector, the withdrawal of supply subsidies forced rents to rise. In so far as low-income tenants received Housing Benefit to cover the full cost of rent, any rises did not adversely affect them. But they did have the effect of ensuring that council housing was made less attractive to medium- and higher-income groups.

Both these developments were accompanied by what has probably become the most internationally renowned piece of housing legislation of the last two decades: the Housing Act 1980. This gave council tenants a right to buy their homes; a right which was backed by large (33–50 per cent) discounts on the market value. By 1989 some 1.15 million households – almost a fifth of the total – had availed themselves of this offer (Department of the Environment, 1991). Much of the 1980s growth of home ownership is thus attributable, firstly, to those who, no longer being able to turn to the public sector because of limited production, sought to meet their housing needs through private provision, and, secondly, to those partaking of the opportunity to buy the home they had previously rented.

For both groups, purchase was facilitated by another set of policies which liberated the mortgage market. This was achieved by ensuring greater competition between banks and building societies, and by removing many of the regulations limiting building society behaviour. One of the developments was the ending of the building society interest rate cartel, which in the 1970s had produced negative real rates of interest, and the consequent raising of interest rates to levels which were positive in real terms. Although this made loans more expensive, it also ensured that mortgage queues no longer constrained the expansion of home ownership.

COMMON OR UNCOMMON DEVELOPMENTS?

In terms of housing policy, as well as in other respects, the Thatcher years are often portrayed as being quite distinctive. But, whatever the distinctiveness of Thatcherism might have been, there are in some important respects continuities over time and space. If what was happening in Britain in the 1980s was not exactly the same as happened in the 1970s, neither was it entirely different. It is also clear that what was happening in Britain in the

1980s was not entirely different from what was happening in a number of other countries. In this section the aim is to identify some of the common and uncommon developments. First, however, it is pertinent to offer some comments about the extent to which the existing literature enables a systematic comparison of developments in European countries.

Before the early part of the 1980s, the literature available in English about housing in European countries other than Britain was limited. David Donnison's *The Government of Housing*, published in 1967, was an early exception which was joined by others such as Headey (1978), Hallett (1977) and Kemeny (1981) only after a decade had elapsed. Although subsequently the literature has mushroomed, its coverage has been geographically uneven. A rough measure of this unevenness is provided by the relative size of each country's membership of the European Network of Housing Researchers which was set up in the mid-1980s. Numerically the membership has been dominated by researchers from three countries – Sweden, the Netherlands and Britain. Germany, France, Belgium and the countries of southern Europe, for example, have been relatively under-represented.

Not only has the geographical coverage been uneven, but what increased research there has been has not dealt exclusively, or even mainly, with home ownership. In part, this reflects the fact that those countries in which housing research has been most active have not themselves had housing systems in which home ownership has played the major part. Sweden, the Netherlands and West Germany have all had housing systems dominated by rental housing. In part it may also reflect a general orientation of housing research towards state policy and social housing. As Michael Ball and his colleagues write:

> Interest in the study of owner-occupied housing markets only evolved in recent years. Before, attention focused on social housing sectors and state housing policies. As such attitudes to research prevailed in most Western countries, a presentation of a cross-national comparison of owner-occupied housing markets on the basis of existing research is very difficult.
>
> (Ball *et al.*, 1988: 87)

So, systematic knowledge of the European experience of home ownership remains incomplete. This pushes comparative statements away both from all European countries or from a predefined group of just two or three countries. In practice, evidence has to be sought where it occurs, which frequently means countries outside Europe – specifically Australia and the USA – in which there is a longer tradition of research interest in home ownership.

The meaning of home ownership

Despite the disparate nature of the country examples, it became increasingly apparent in the 1980s that studies of comparative housing systems commonly share a definitional problem. Whereas all Western countries have a form of housing which is labelled 'home ownership' (and equally other forms labelled 'private rental' and 'social housing'), the label does not necessarily refer to the same phenomenon. There is, in other words, a 'gap between the taxonomic collective and the substantial reality' (Barlow and Duncan, 1988: 225). Thus the nature of what is being described can change, so that 'to generalise about owner occupation is to categorise unlike things together' (Ball, 1986:157). The unlikeness can occur over time, as Forrest and Murie (1983) suggest, after Fred Hirsch, that the expansion of home ownership in Britain may lead to its dilution as a positional good, so that the status derived from the ownership of this scarce good wanes as it becomes less scarce. In that sense the position of a home owner in Britain in 1960 may have been very different from the position of the owner of the same house in 1990.

The unlikeness may be greater between countries. A characteristic of home ownership in Finland, for example, is that much of it takes the organisational form of the housing company in which there may be pooling, amongst the individual shareholders, of costs and facilities, such as laundry and sauna. In addition, much home ownership in Finland can be described as social housing, since access to subsidised housing loans has been means tested and the maximum cost of the housing limited (see Ruonavaara, 1987). In the United States, on the other hand, home ownership has often taken the physical form of the mobile home. Indeed, in 1972 mobile homes accounted for one-third of all new, single-family housing. Because they have a short life expectancy, and in any case are not considered to be real estate, available loans for their purchase are generally short term and with high interest rates. Unlike many other forms of home ownership in other countries, their exchange value falls rapidly over time (Ball *et al.*, 1988). In Sweden, most home ownership is produced under forms of state regulation and support, with construction companies building to local authority specifications on local authority land (Barlow and Duncan, 1988). In West Germany, much home ownership has been self-promoted, usually through contracting a private builder, by higher-income groups aged in their 30s or older (Barlow and Duncan, 1988). Such examples show that, from one country to another, home ownership's meaning for individual owners, in terms of cost, access, built-form, lifestyle, status, and so on, can vary considerably. In considering home ownership, therefore, there must be a recognition that whilst it may be tempting to think of a homogeneous and constant phenomenon that can be defined in terms of what Hindess (1987) refers to as 'the essentialism of the market', there may actually be significant variations over time and space.

Long-term growth in Britain

Notwithstanding such variations, in terms of numbers the growth in home ownership in Britain in the 1980s was not the growth of a tenure that had previously been static in size. At the start of the century about 10 per cent of households had been owners. The favourable tax treatment of home owners, the continued development of the building societies and the growth in real incomes all contributed to the growth of the sector to about 30 per cent by 1950. Although there were large programmes of council house building, particularly in the early post-war years, each decade after 1950 experienced a small, steady growth in the proportion of home owners. The distinctiveness of the 1980s, therefore, was not that home ownership expanded, but that, in part at least as a result of deliberate encouragement by government, its rate of expansion accelerated. It was the speed of growth rather than growth itself which was different. Depending upon developments in the 1990s, the 1980s may in retrospect be seen either as a period of acceleration or as a temporary surge in an underlying trend.

Growth elsewhere

The British experience was also not uncommon in the sense that home ownership expanded in many Western countries in the post-war period. Between 1950 and 1980 the average annual rate of expansion of home ownership in the countries recorded in Table 4.1 was highest – by far – in the UK, but the rate was also relatively high in Italy and Austria, and positive in all of them. Consequently, whereas in 1950 the average percentage size of home ownership over the 14 countries recorded was 40 per cent, by 1980 the average had risen to 54 per cent. So a greater reliance on home ownership as a means of meeting housing needs has been a common feature of post-war Europe.

However, Table 4.1 also shows that any general trend has actually been far from uniform in outcome. The rates of growth were positive for all the countries for which data were recorded, but they were relatively low in some countries – Sweden and Denmark, for example – and indeed actually fell in some countries in some decades. Evidence of the large differences between countries in the extent to which their home-owning sectors have grown was in fact presented at the outset of the 1980s.

Kemeny (1981) distinguished between two groups of countries. The English-speaking countries of Australia, Canada, New Zealand and the

Table 4.1 Annual rate of growth of percentage of stock in home ownership
1950–80

Country	Annual rate of growth (%)
Austria	1.3
Belgium	1.1
Denmark	0.3
Finland	0.4
France	0.9
Ireland	1.2
Italy	1.5
Netherlands	1.2
Norway	1.2
Sweden	0.3
Switzerland	1.0
UK	2.4
USA	0.8
West Germany	1.1

Source: Calculated from data given in UN, *Annual Bulletin of Housing and Building Statistics for Europe.*

USA, he argued, all have housing systems based on private forms of provision. With a low percentage of their stocks consisting of welfare housing, the main parts are divided between private renting (25–35 per cent) and home owning (60–70 per cent). There is a second group of countries – the Netherlands, Sweden, Switzerland and West Germany, for example – which have developed large cost-rental alternatives to home owning. In these countries the size of the home-owning sectors has increased during at least some of the the post-war years, but their relative size remains small. Notwithstanding Kemeny's omission of a number of European countries – in particular Norway and Finland – which have high home ownership rates, Britain stands out as an odd case in this particular classification since it has both a large home-owning sector *and* a large cost-rental (council) sector. Interestingly, the 1980s was a decade in which Britain, as a result of council house sales, was moving away from the cost-rental countries towards the home-owning ones. In this sense, therefore, Britain has been moving *away* from the European model, with its main comparators now to be found in North America and Australasia.

Accounting for common and uncommon developments

One view is that the greater reliance in many countries on home ownership can be understood as one element of wider processes of housing privatisation, although this does not mean that privatisation and home ownership are necessarily linked. Nevertheless, the typical post-war response had been social housing provision and extensive regulation, summarised by Wollmann and Jaedicke(1989: 82): 'faced with an enormous housing shortage in the immediate post war years, in most Western countries housing policy was characterised by a high degree of state intervention. The entire housing sector was put, to a considerable extent, under public guidance and control.'

Some forms of withdrawal of state intervention occurred within only a few years; for example, the relaxation of building licences in 1950s' Britain, and the increased reliance on private provision in France and Germany (see the individual country chapters in Wynn, 1984, for post-war policy developments in a number of European countries). However, the major moves towards privatisation of housing (as well as other areas of welfare) occurred from the late 1960s onwards. In Tosics' view (Tosics, 1987) this characteristically occurred in two stages. The first stage occurred in the context of the development of housing surpluses (or at least housing shortages had virtually come to an end) and of buoyant economies. It consisted of a redirection of subsidies from production (subsidised rents) to demand (tax and rent allowances). In this stage, therefore, the emphasis was shifted from general assistance through costs, towards individual assistance through incomes. The second stage, occurring from the mid-1970s onwards, 'can be considered as a consequence of economic followed by political-ideological changes, which were independent of the housing sector'(Tosics, 1987: 65). In this stage 'the participation of the state in the housing sector is decreasing ... and it is also biased toward assisting private ownership' (1987: 66).

British council house sales perhaps provide the stereotype for Tosics' stage two; indeed they provided an exemplar for privatisation in one of the countries that, in tenure trends, Britain was itself emulating. Thus Silver (1990: 123) notes that:

The privatization of American low-income housing programs in general, and the sale of public housing in particular, long preceded the Reagan Administration. Yet the apparent success of Mrs Thatcher's 'right to buy' policy ... gave the policy new impetus in the United States during the 1980s. Responding to the advocates from New Right think tanks and citing the British experience, the President's Commission on Housing proposed public housing sales in its 1982 report.

Nevertheless, as a generalisation, the description of the two stages disguises considerable international variation; to the extent that the usefulness of a *stages of development* type explanation becomes doubtful. In Australia, for example, the main policy developments in stage two have been the deregulation of financial institutions (Carter, 1990) rather than the sale of public housing as in Britain. In the Netherlands, by contrast, the Van Agt cabinet of 1977–81 set out programmes for curbing state expenditure on housing and encouraging sales of privately rented housing and the extension of home ownership. Within a few years, increasing unemployment and rising mortgage interest rates combined with a home ownership market which was showing signs of excess supply. In these circumstances 'what could the buyer-friendly cabinet do?' (Priemus, 1987: 22). Whatever the possibilities, the government actually responded with a policy of what might be called de-privatisation, involving increasing subsidies to rental housing production. So, in the case of the Netherlands, there was a reversion from stage two to stage one. Even for Britain it has been argued that, rather than state participation *decreasing* in stage two, it has been restructured. The withdrawal of subsidies from local authority housing has been more than offset by increases in tax benefits to home owners. Forrest and Murie (1988) have coined the phrase 'subsidised individualism' to describe a shifts toward support for home ownership which is not divorcing the state from the housing system, but which is rather a reorientation of state intervention.

The recognition of this degree of cross-national variation around a putative norm is important because of a strong tradition in housing research. It is perhaps a testament to the influence of David Donnison's 1967 book that Barnett *et al.* (1985) were able to claim that a high proportion of comparative housing research had been founded, explicitly or implicitly, on notions of convergence and stages of development. Applied to tenure developments, these notions would be that levels of home ownership were a function of economic development, and that they would become increasingly similar over time. However, not only has diversity, rather than similarity, been established above by reference to individual country cases, but other recent research has cast considerable doubt on the usefulness of this type of explanation. At a broad level it has been rejected in two studies which have tested a convergence theory explanation of housing developments (Schmidt, 1989; Doling, 1990c). On the basis of the statistical indicators used there is little support for views that housing systems are becoming increasingly similar; indeed, the evidence for divergence seems somewhat stronger (see also Kemeny, forthcoming).

An alternative explanatory avenue has been explored by Kemeny (1981) with his suggestion that the political influence of socialist parties in each country has been positively related to the extent to which welfare housing has been developed. However, his conclusion that 'it is important not to overestimate party-political differences in terms of tenure policy' (p. 63) has been endorsed, in what is perhaps the only systematic test of this hypothesis, with the statement that 'it seems unlikely that socialist parties throughout the industrialised countries pursue a common distinct policy with respect to tenure' (Schmidt, 1989: 94).

Home ownership and ideology

The position we have reached so far, then, is that cross-national similarities and differences with regard to trends in the taxonomic collective cannot adequately be explained either by a convergence/stages of development thesis or by a political parties in power thesis. A more promising approach might be one centred on 'society's welfare ideological orientation' (Schmidt, 1989: 94). The empirical significance of this approach rests on a very marked correlation ($r = -0.88$) to be found between levels of home ownership and degrees of 'welfare collectivism' (as measured by levels of family allowances, pensions, sickness benefits, unemployment support, etc. as a percentage of total public expenditure). In other words, those countries that have a strong commitment towards welfare collectivism tend to have housing systems that emphasise forms of collective, rental housing, whereas those with a so-called 'weaker welfare collectivism commitment' place more emphasis upon individualised home ownership (see Figure 4.1). This is of course a categorisation which merely locates countries along a continuum irrespective of *types* of welfare commitment (see other typologies present and referred to in this volume). Furthermore Schmidt himself warns that the 'relationship should not be interpreted in a narrow manner, that is to say, as a simple cause and effect model' (1989: 95). He adds:

> It is not very likely that the scope of public welfare determines the structure of the housing market, or vice versa. Rather, observations suggest that the structure of the housing market is affected by the same factors as public welfare in general. . . . Both public welfare (or lack of it) and tenure forms are expressions for more fundamental social values concerning the appropriate balance between public/collective and private/individual spheres.
>
> (Schmidt, 1989: 95)

This suggests that countries may have deeper and more enduring ideological bases, which may transcend general elections, which may themselves alter the balance of seats held by right- and left-wing politicians. In those countries with high levels of home ownership, the ideological base may incorporate life goals centred on the achievement of home ownership. Such a life goal has been described for Finland, for example, by Hannu Ruonavaara (1988). They may find expression in catchphrases about the desirability of home owning. Schmidt refers to 'the Great Australian Dream'

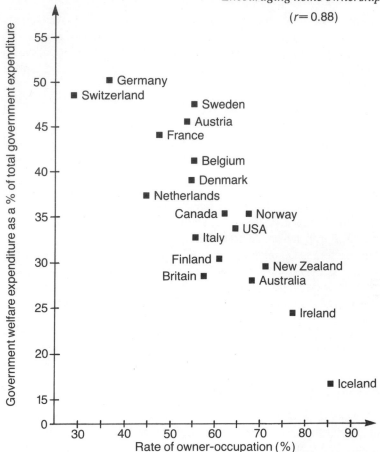

Figure 4.1 Relationship between government welfare expenditure (percentage of total government expenditure) and the relative size of the owner-occupied sector (mid-1980s)
Source: Schmidt (1989).

and 'the American Way of Life', to which might be added 'the Englishman's Home is his Castle'. The importance of home ownership in the British culture has been commented upon by Peter Saunders (1990: 40):

> The popularity of the twentieth century tenurial revolution in Britain is testimony to the strength of 800 years of a cultural tradition which is distinctive from that of mainland Europe. This is not to suggest that continental European cultures do not also carry strong individualistic values, nor that their peoples have not desired their own homes. Before the First World War, for example, German factory workers apparently

'yearned' for small private houses of their own. . . . However, only around 40 per cent of the West German population has even today fulfilled this yearning, and this does suggest that the desire for individual private property may run deeper in English culture than it does in the German.

Notwithstanding Saunders' over-generalisation about the similarity of cultures in the countries of mainland Europe, his argument can be related to our earlier comments concerning tenure strategies. National cultures might be thought of as having guided policy development such that, independent of the political leanings of parties in government, structures have been established which encourage the pursuit of life goals. The structures may both encourage the growth of home ownership and, in so doing, reinforce the ideology. In some countries the ideology finds expression in home ownership, but in others different ideology encourages an orientation to other tenure forms. On this view, the long-term growth of home ownership in Britain has been founded on an ideology supporting this tenure form, which has been an enduring feature of much of the present century. Although the strength of the ideology waned during some periods, notably in the immediate post-war years, the significance of the 1980s was that the political and the underlying ideological structure developed and came together in a particular way which gave impetus to home ownership.

HOUSING CRISES IN THE 1980s

So far we have provided evidence that Britain is not alone in achieving a high rate of home ownership. Neither is it alone in having an ideology which finds expression in a tenure form which may vary from country to country in a number of ways but which shares a taxonomic label. Reliance upon market provision, in the form of home ownership, rather than state provision, however, means that the housing circumstances of individuals become susceptible to the dynamics of a number of interrelated markets in labour, finance and housing. Although the exact nature of these dynamics varies across countries, increasingly there is evidence that the growth of home-owning sectors has been accompanied by difficulties in many countries. So, whatever the ideological foundation of increasing home ownership, economic developments may act as an effective limit on that increase. Gaps in the literature prevent the presentation of a comprehensive picture, but it is apparent that the home ownership markets of the 1980s have sometimes proved problematic such that individual difficulties have accumulated to create market-wide crises.

Affordability

One of the results, at least in part, of the privatisation of housing in Britain has been that 'for most consumers, housing became more expensive in the 1980s' (Kleinman and Whitehead, 1988: 16). This experience holds for a number of other countries, where there have been general trends in the direction of increased costs of entry into home ownership. This may have occurred because house prices have continued to increase over the long run, though as we discuss in a later section the experience differs between countries, and there may be short-run decreases. However, a further increase in costs, and one which is directly related to policy developments, has occurred in at least some of those countries that have deregulated their financial markets. Some countries that had housing finance circuits in which loans for housing were rationed by bureaucratic rules that entailed queuing have established systems in which loans are rationed through price. In Britain (Kleinman and Whitehead, 1988), Australia and New Zealand (Thorns, 1988), Finland (Doling, 1990b), Greece (Emmanuel, 1990) and Southern Ireland (Blackwell, 1990), for example, such developments have resulted in interest rates, which had been negative in real terms, becoming positive in real terms in the 1980s. While in Britain the combined effect of central government policy has been to make access to home ownership easier, access has nevertheless been 'at a somewhat higher cost for the majority' (Kleinman and Whitehead, 1988: 9). In both Australia and New Zealand, by contrast, 'the purchase of a property has consequently consumed an increasing proportion of household income and made access to owner-occupation increasingly difficult for lower income households' (Thorns, 1988: 72). So in some countries households entering home ownership have been required to pay higher costs for borrowing money, and this may itself be establishing upper limits to the growth of this tenure form.

Mortgage default

One of the common, though not essential, characteristics of home ownership is that it entails households committing themselves to large loans, in relation to income, which are repaid over extensive periods of time. However, in many respects, Western countries have become more uncertain or risky environments in which to make large and long-term financial commitments. Large increases in unemployment, in household break-up rates and in interest rate volatility mean that budgetary arrangements are vulnerable. The result for house buyers is sometimes that their willingness and ability to meet housing costs are reduced. The changing structures of housing systems with more emphasis on private provision, therefore, are structures within which financial difficulty may become more likely, and this has consequences for the ability of home owners to maintain their housing position.

In Britain in the 1980s, decreases in income, together with increases in housing and non-housing costs, have resulted in large increases in levels of default on building society mortgages. Over the period 1979–85, levels of default increased by about sixfold. One estimate is that, by the mid-1980s, 5 per cent of all building society borrowers were at least the equivalent of two monthly payments in arrears (Doling *et al.*, 1988). Following a reduction in arrears in the period 1986–88, they have subsequently risen even higher: perhaps to 6 per cent of borrowers (Ford, 1989). The immediate cause of this latest increase was a rapid hike in interest rates from about 10 per cent in 1988 to 15 per cent in 1990.

But mortgage default is by no means confined to Britain. It has long been a feature of the housing market in the USA (see Gellen, 1977, for an early review). By the early 1980s default had reached a then record 5.4 per cent of all borrowers (Dreier, 1982). The 1980s also provided evidence that default can reach significant levels even where, as in the case of West Germany, home ownership tends to be confined to higher-income groups (Potter and Drevermann, 1988). Here the conjunction of the particular subsidy structure, low wage inflation, high loan/income ratios and labour market difficulties led to foreclosure proceedings doubling from 1980 to 1986. In this West German case the rather undeveloped second-hand market, and the conditions imposed by the lending institutions to protect their investment, frequently mean that buyers have left home ownership with large debts. In contrast, there is evidence that default is at insignificant levels in Finland even though rates of both home ownership and unemployment are at high levels. This appears largely to result from a combination of the high average age of the unemployed, who thus have low average levels of housing debt, and the presence of supportive financial institutions and social security systems (Doling, 1990a). Mortgage default is not, therefore, a universal phenomenon even where unemployment levels appear to be unfavourable.

House prices

Although in the long run house prices in Britain have increased, there have been short-run changes in house prices. Thus in those periods and places where house buyers have experienced reduced incomes or higher costs, the ability and willingness of households to maintain their mortgage commitments or to move up market and take on larger commitments have been affected. In fact the experience in Britain has been that the opposite occurs: people move out of home ownership or down market, transactions slump and prices fall (Doling and Koskiaho, 1990). In the 1980s prices fell – in money as well as in real terms – during the period 1981–82 when unemployment was increasing most rapidly, and again during 1988–90 when interest rates rose most quickly. There were also important geographical variations. In the first period the falls were greatest in those parts of the country – the Midlands and the North – where unemployment was greatest, and in the second period in the South where loan/income ratios were highest (Doling and Ford, 1991). There has been some discussion about whether regional divergences in prices have been temporary trends or part of a long-term restructuring of British housing markets (see Hamnett, 1988).

As with mortgage default, short-run slumps in housing markets and regional price variations are not confined to Britain. In the case of Finland for instance, prices in the 1980s increased rapidly in those parts of the country – particularly the south around the capital, Helsinki – which were expanding economically, and decreased relatively in those parts which were declining economically (Doling and Koskiaho, 1990). During the first years of the 1980s, house prices in many other West European countries – the Netherlands, West Germany, France, Sweden, Denmark – as well as the USA were depressed (Ball *et al.*, 1988; Duncan, 1990). In all of these countries, falling house prices can alter the attractiveness of home ownership by modifying its investment characteristics, to the effect that both individual households and financial institutions may be less willing to invest in housing.

FUTURE PROSPECTS

In terms of apparent policy objectives – a shift from public to private provision, particularly in the form of home ownership – the policy instruments selected by the British government in the 1980s have achieved considerable success. Nevertheless, in a number of other respects the housing experiences of British home owners are problematic. Affordability problems and mortgage default are at record levels, which together with short-run price developments perhaps indicate a market currently at the limits of its growth potential. Although policy is orientated in such a way as to increase home ownership, and although this is consistent with ideological predilections, growth may not be sustainable in the future. In that sense the ideological has come up against the economic. Furthermore, while there are differences from country to country – as we have indicated – in levels of default and price decreases, much about the British experience is not unique.

In these common experiences there is a paradox. One of the cornerstones of the restructuring of welfare states in the 1970s and 1980s has been the changing economic conditions, which have proved fertile breeding grounds for the development of neo-liberal policies. Continuing economic difficulties have created a context, however, in which the policy outcomes have proved problematic. Although it would of course be naive to suggest that the development of problems within national housing systems will automatically be translated into ameliorative action by national governments, they may have an indirect effect by undermining the privatisation/home-owning hegemony. This might, in turn, lead to political demands for new initiatives and/or the possibility of changes in the parties in power. Consequently, it is legitimate to consider what forms policy developments in the 1990s might take.

1 *Keeping the same course.* In this scenario, some Western governments may retain their existing policy frameworks with minimal change. If the objective is to increase private provision, however, the impact of existing policies alone may be limited. Thus in Britain, despite the early success in boosting the numbers of home owners, there was by the end of the decade a realisation within government 'that there is an upper limit to the spread of home ownership [so that] probably at least 25–30 per cent of households will be tenants at any one time' (Kleinman, 1990: 94). In fact, this seems to be consistent with the general experience of home ownership in Western countries. Thus in Australia, New Zealand and the USA home ownership rates had reached levels in excess of two-thirds before the onset of the 1970s, but have not subsequently increased. Indeed, in the case of the USA the rate has decreased. Although the differing nature of home ownership and the differing market structures in different countries militate against the proposition of a universal law governing the size of home-owning sectors, nevertheless there is evidence, as we have shown, that the limits of growth under present arrangements are sometimes being exposed.

2 *Further privatisation.* Some governments may introduce further privatisation measures. These could follow Tosics' suggestion that the logic of the present arguments against state intervention would result in a 'third stage' in which such subsidies to owners (for example, in the form of tax relief on mortgage interest payments) were also withdrawn (Tosics, 1987). This would be consistent with the policy initiatives proposed by neo-liberal writers who see tax relief as an undesirable intervention.

3 *De-privatisation.* Difficulties encountered with home ownership may lead some governments to re-establish support for social housing. Thus, instead of moving on from Tosics' stage two to stage three, it would constitute a step back to stage one.

4 *Support for existing home ownership.* This could take the form of social security benefits for home owners who face financial difficulties, perhaps by extending housing allowances to low-income owners. It might also be a recognition that the private provision of housing worked

most smoothly where it was sustained by public action. Given the continuation of economic difficulties, the question of resources might be resolved by combining policy options (2) and (4). This would constitute a redistribution of subsidy from home buyers in general (though the incidence of subsidy has generally been weighted toward higher-income groups) to low-income buyers.

The precise effect any of these developments might have on the size of home ownership sectors is unknown. O'sullivan's assessment of the state of knowledge of the housing finance system in Britain – 'that no full scenario of its effects is currently available' (O'sulllivan, 1984: 141) – can be applied more or less equally to other countries. Nevertheless we can speculate that under option (4) home ownership will increase, under (2) and (3) decrease, and under (1) remain static or increase slightly. Significantly, these are not options likely to be affected in the short to medium term by the impact of the Single Market, the provisions of the Social Chapter or other moves in the direction of EC harmonisation. However, there may in future be increased awareness, on the part of individual national social housing organisations, of practices being followed elsewhere.

REFERENCES

Ball, M. (1986) 'Housing analysis: time for a theoretical refocus', *Housing Studies* 1, 147–65.

Ball M., Harloe, M. and Martens, M. (1988) *Housing and Social Change in Europe and the USA*, London: Routledge.

Barlow, J. and Duncan, S. (1988) 'The use and abuse of housing tenure', *Housing Studies* 3, (4), 219–31.

Barnett, I., Groth, A. J. and Ungson, C. (1985) 'East–west housing policies', in A. J. Groth and L. Wade (eds) *Public Housing across Nations*, Greenwich, Conn.: JAI Press.

Blackwell, J. (1990) 'Housing finance and subsidies in Ireland', in D. Maclennan and R. Williams (eds) *Affordable Housing in Europe*, York: Joseph Rowntree Foundation.

Carter, R.A. (1990) 'Mortgage-backed securities, inflation-adjusted mortgages, and real-rate funding: recent initiatives in housing finance in Australia', in W. van Vliet and J. van Weesep (eds) *Government and Housing: Developments in Seven Countries*, Newbury Park: Sage.

Department of the Environment (1991) *Housing and Construction Statistics*, London: HMSO.

Doling, J. (1990a) 'Mortgage default: why Finland is not like Britain', *Environment and Planning A* 22, 321–31.

—— (1990b) 'Housing finance in Finland', in D. Maclennan and R. Williams (eds) *Affordable Housing in Europe*, York: Joseph Rowntree Foundation.

—— (1990c) 'Housing policy and convergence theory: some comments on Schmidt', *Scandinavian Housing and Planning Research* 7, 117–20.

Doling, J. and Ford, J. (1991) 'The changing face of home ownership: building societies and household investment strategies', *Policy and Politics*, 19, 109–18.

Doling, J. and Koskiaho, B. (1990) 'Economic restructuring, intranational house price changes and social security: the case of Britain and Finland', *Scandinavian Housing and Planning Research* 7, 3–15.

Doling, J., Ford, J. and Stafford, B. (1988) *The Property Owing Democracy*, Aldershot: Gower.

Donnison, D. (1967) *The Government of Housing*, Harmondsworth: Penguin.

Dreier, P. (1982) 'The housing crisis: dreams and nightmares', *The Nation*, August, 21–8.

Duncan, S.S. (1990) 'Do house prices rise that much? A dissenting view', *Housing Studies* 5, 195–208.

Emmanuel, D. (1990) 'Housing finance in Greece', in D. Maclennan and R. Williams (eds) *Affordable Housing in Europe*, York: Joseph Rowntree Foundation.

Ford, J. (1989) 'Pity the poor home owners – again', *Roof* 14, 6.

Forrest, R. and Murie, A. (1983) 'Residualisation and council housing: aspects of the changing social relations of housing', *Journal of Social Policy* 12 (4), 452–68.

—— (1988) *Selling the welfare state*, London: Routledge.

Gellen, M. (1977) *The Cause of Mortgage Foreclosure: A Review of the Literature*, Working Paper 279/MFS–02, Institute of Urban and Regional Development, University of California, Berkeley.

Hallett, G. (1977) *Housing and Land Policies in West Germany and Britain*, Basingstoke: Macmillan.

Hamnett, C. (1988) 'Regional variations in house prices and house price inflation in Britain 1969–1988', *Royal Bank of Scotland Review*, no. 159, 29–40.

Headey, B. (1978) *Housing Policy in the Developed Economy*, London: Croom Helm.

Hindess, B. (1987) *Freedom, Equality and the Market: Arguments on Social Policy*, Tavistock Press.

Kemeny, J. (1981) *The Myth of Home Ownership*, London: Routledge & Kegan Paul.

—— (forthcoming) *Housing and Social Theory*, London: Routledge.

Kleinman, M. (1990) 'The future provision of rental housing in Britain', in W. van Vliet and J. van Weesep (eds) *Government and Housing: Developments in Seven Countries*, Newbury Park: Sage.

Kleinman, M. and Whitehead, C. (1988) 'British housing since 1979: has the system changed?' *Housing Studies*, 3, 3–19.

Malpass, P. (1990) *Reshaping Housing Policy: Subsidies, Rents and Residualisation*, London: Routledge.

O'Sullivan, A. (1984) 'Misconceptions in the current housing subsidy debate', *Policy and Politics* 12, 119–44.

Potter, P. and Drevermann, M. (1988) 'Home ownership, foreclosure and compulsory auction in the Federal Republic of Germany', *Housing Studies* 3, 94–104.

Priemus, H. (1987) 'Economic and demographic stagnation, housing and housing policy', *Housing Studies* 2, 17–27.

Ruonavaara, H. (1987) 'The Kemeny approach: the case of Finland', *Scandinavia Housing and Planning Research* 4, 163–77.

—— (1988) *The Growth of Urban Home-Ownership in Finland 1950–1980*, University of Turku, Department of Sociology and Political Research, Sociological Studies Series A No. 10.

Saunders, P. (1990) *A Nation of Home Owners*, London: Allen & Unwin.

Schmidt, S. (1989) 'Convergence theory, labour movements, and corporatism: the case of housing', *Scandinavian Housing and Planning Research* 6, 83–101.

Silver, H. (1990) 'Privatizsation, self-help, and public-housing home ownership in the United States', in W. van Vliet and J. van Weesep (eds) *Government and Housing: Developments in Seven Countries*, Newbury Park: Sage.

Thorns, D. (1988) 'New solutions to old problems: housing affordability and access within Australia and New Zealand', *Environment and Planning A* 20, 71–82.

Tosics, I. (1987) 'Privatization in housing policy: the case of Western countries and Hungary', *International Journal of Urban and Regional Research* 11, 61–77.

Wollmann, H. and Jaedicke, W. (1989) 'The rise and fall of public and social housing', *Tijdschrift voor economische en sociale geografie* 80, 82–8.

Wynn, M. (1984) *Housing in Europe*, London: Croom Helm.

Young, H. (1983) Interview with Mrs Thatcher, *Sunday Times*, 27 February, p 29.

5 Privatism and partnership in urban policy
Some comparative issues

Nicholas Deakin

INTRODUCTION

This essay reviews some recent developments in British urban policy, with particular emphasis on the extent to which the policy-making process has had a comparative dimension. In practice, this has meant almost exclusively the exchange of ideas and experience between Britain and the United States.

Thus, when about to set out on one of the frequent visits that he and his ministerial colleagues have made to the United States in search of lessons for inner-city policy, Kenneth Clarke – who was then minister in charge of the British urban regeneration programme – commented that 'the US is the only country in the world from which Britain has anything to learn in tackling inner city problems' (1988a). Clarke was not alone in this belief. Numerous academic specialists in urban policy have followed the same trail over the past two decades. To justify this process, Hambleton (1990) points to a series of developments common to both countries, which he regards as particularly significant: growing internal disparities in prosperity within the two countries; rapid decline (as part of that process) of older cities whose economic base rested on the prosperity of manufacturing industry; growing social polarisation within those cities; and attempts by city authorities, in mutual competition, to revive their economies by measures designed to attract new investment.

But in fact none of these developments has been exclusive to Anglo-Saxon countries. If there are common factors that unite Britain and the United States they might be more plausibly located in the mutual failures of many past policy interventions, in both analysis and execution. And these failures in turn derive (I would suggest) at least in part from misunderstanding or misuse of the common experience of the two countries (Rose, 1974) – and in the British case an unwillingness to draw on other experience.

This unwillingness – and, in particular, the reluctance of UK policy

makers, at all levels, to draw lessons from developments in the rest of Europe
– might well be thought odd. There are good reasons for believing that a
convergence in experience is in the course of taking place, as policy makers
throughout the European Community find themselves facing a common
agenda of pressing issues, on which urban problems command a prominent
place. This process will undoubtedly be hastened by current moves towards
a closer alignment of social policies as the Community moves towards closer
political and economic unity. In some policy areas the importance of
understanding and learning from the experience in the rest of Europe is
already well understood – witness the evangelising labours of John Stewart
and Michael Clarke in seeking to interest colleagues in the British local
authority world in different experimental models of local government in the
rest of Europe (see Stewart and Clarke, 1990). Comparative research to
support these endeavours is still at an early stage in its development; but the
creation of new networks of academic specialists is entering a phase of
exponential growth. Why, then, have policy makers been slow to pick up the
cue?

Two reasons might be suggested: first, ideological incompatibilities and,
second, other cultural and (whisper it) even linguistic differences. The first
is specific to the 1980s, when both Britain and the United States elected
governments of the right committed to market-based policies, which had a
particularly sharp impact on the urban policy field. Despite widespread
interest amongst the rest of the European Community in the policies being
adopted, there was never any real question, as the title of a particularly
hyperbolic text of the mid-1980s proclaimed, of Britain's example
'privatising the world'. Under a thin topdressing of rhetoric, governments
elsewhere continued to play a central part in policy making and
implementation regardless of the new Anglo-Saxon passion for reducing the
role of the state. This divergence provided one ingredient in the policy
conflicts of the late 1980s and in Margaret Thatcher's stubborn – and
ultimately (for her) fatal – resistance to the concept of a more interventionist
role for Brussels.

The other reason that might have been responsible for lack of interest in
European models was that many of the techniques associated with the new
urban policies adopted in Britain were of American origin – new approaches
to management dating back to planned programme and budget systems of
the 1960s and evolving from them into a succession of new techniques, all
designed to transform the nature of the public services by importing skills
and experience from the private sector. In practice, the long shadow of the
business schools (in which many of these techniques were nurtured and
developed) has also fallen over European public administration; an MBA
(and competence in English) is increasingly common among ambitious

young administrators. But the sense has been that, in terms of the culture of the public sector, Europe has little to teach but much to learn.

Whatever the reasons, the outcome has been clear: the basis for comparison and exchange has been and remains transatlantic, not cross-Channel.

SOME ANGLO-AMERICAN ATTITUDES

The transatlantic dialogue on urban policy issues over the post-war period has been punctuated by a series of formal gatherings of various kinds involving politicians, practitioners, academics and on occasion volatile mixtures of all three. One favourite location for these exchanges has been Ditchley Park (the more than stately home of the Anglo-American Foundation) and it was here that one of the more celebrated gatherings took place at the end of October 1969.

References to this Ditchley Conference abound in the British litera-ture on urban regeneration (Marris, 1982; Hambleton, 1991; Community Development Projects, 1977a, b, etc.). Reading the transcript of proceedings today, it is hard to see anything to justify some of the conspiratorial interpretations subsequently placed upon it, notably by the Community Development Projects (CDP) teams whose future activities were one of the topics under review. True, its parentage was suspect – the agreement by President Nixon and Prime Minister Wilson 'to look together at social and economic issues affecting our two societies'. But whatever the two men's subsequent reputation – posterity has not, so far, been kind – it is hard to see anything deeply sinister in the modest calls for more research and better evaluation that punctuated proceedings or in the Chairman's traditional closing wish that the Conference should be treated as a 'starting point, not an end of dialogue' (Anglo-American Conference on Experiments in Social Policy, 1969, p. 43).

Yet there is one sense in which the subsequent notoriety of the October 1969 gathering is justified. It came at a time when the policy community in the United States was bidding farewell to an attempt to address urban decline through systematic intervention by the federal government – the Great Society programmes of President Lyndon Johnson and complex of social policy initiatives propelled by the civil rights movement of the 1960s that made up the War on Poverty. Many of the veterans of this struggle who attended the Ditchley gathering were suffering from combat fatigue and some had become a shade cynical. In any case, President Nixon's recent election gave little grounds for supposing that combat could be continued on the terms and level of commitment set by the Johnson administration. Moreover, there was by 1969 a more than slight suspicion that the outcome would be – in a phrase used at Ditchley by one participant (English, as it happens) and subsequently picked up by outside critics – merely to 'gild the ghetto'.

Within five years of the Ditchley gathering the British experiment, the Community Development Projects, though conducted on an infinitely smaller scale and with far more limited aspirations, had also run into the sands (Higgins, Deakin, Edwards and Wicks, 1983; Loney, 1983). The teams established in a dozen small areas to focus community-based effort on combating urban decay had rapidly reached the conclusion that the real location of the problems that those areas faced lay elsewhere, in structural changes in the national (if not global) economy and in the policies adopted by central government to deal with them. Repudiated by their parent government department (the Home Office), the teams went out in a splutter of critical reports defiantly declaring their belief in the futility of locally based action (Marris, 1982; CDP, 1977a, b).

The sense of failure left by these successive episodes on both sides of the Atlantic lingered on, as did the impression that the British had made an important strategic error in calling upon American models for social action at the precise moment when the Americans themselves were in the course of abandoning them (see A.H. Halsey's crack about ideas drifting across the Atlantic from West to East to be cast up 'soggy on arrival'). Nevertheless, the issues themselves remained on the policy agenda – benign neglect was never a practicable option. Alternative policies to address the problems of urban decline and its impact on inner-city populations were accordingly devised in both countries in the late 1970s.

Although parallel in time, this change in the direction of policies took different forms in the two countries. But policy makers in both countries had in common a determination to move away from the discredited approaches of the immediate past. Specifically, they rejected a reliance on social programmes targeted on small areas to deliver substantial benefits to local populations. Contrary to some subsequent stereotypes, these changes in policy direction towards urban regeneration were not initially the product of the New Right regimes that subsequently came to power in both countries; they were the responsibility of the Carter administration in the United States and the Callaghan government in Britain.

The Carter approach took as its point of departure the 'New Federalism' of his predecessor Richard Nixon, which was in turn based on the assumption that one clear lesson of the 1960s was that urban regeneration (social or economic) could not be achieved through direct executive intervention by the federal government. The core of the new approach consisted of a 'new partnership' between government at all levels and the private sector, designed principally to promote local economic development.

The emphasis would be not on subsidising costly social programmes but on stimulating demand for labour through job creation. To achieve this, the President's Urban and Regional Policy Group (1978) came up with a package of proposals: the creation of a new Urban Development Action Grant (UDAG) administered by Housing and Urban Development (HUD) and designed to subsidise new private investment in inner urban areas; an Economic Development Agency to support and promote locally based Development Corporations with quasi-public status and a new generation of tax-exempt bonds to be issued by state and local governments to provide the financial basis for new private sector development. The whole package was to be held together by new civic leadership in which the local private sector would be a key partner. Although this programme was much reduced in scope by Congress, its outlines were still clearly visible in subsequent policy developments under Carter's successor, Ronald Reagan, elected in 1980.

An especially significant element in the Carter programme was the revival of enthusiasm for and by the private sector, which had been dampened by the experience of the Johnson years. Barnekov and colleagues (on whose account I have leant heavily) comment that, in the late 1960s, 'the enthusiasm for business activism in seeking solutions to the problems of poverty and racism was rapidly drained once the threat of urban violence subsided and the experience with corporate programmes had demonstrated the limits of 'business knowhow''(1989: 60). With the new directions in policy adopted after 1978, the role of the business sector developed along more familiar and comfortable lines which helped to make participation in partnership less problematic.

The changes that took place in Britain over the same period also laid stress on the key significance of economic revival as the engine of change in the inner city and proposed partnership as the means of promoting it; but this was to be a partnership between the different levels of government. Peter Shore as Secretary of State for the Environment in the Callaghan government promoted this approach in his White Paper, *Policy for the Inner Cities* (HMSO, 1977). The White Paper proposed a concentration of resources on seven major inner-city areas in which formal partnerships were created; three-year rolling programmes for regeneration were to be drawn up, with funding from the government's Urban Programme (in a revamped form of the original special grant first devised in 1969) and also from resources produced by 'bending' mainstream programmes. The emphasis on promoting economic regeneration was backed by proposals for the involvement of both private sector and local inhabitants, though strictly in a supporting role.

In several important respects, the programmes adopted in the two countries in the late 1970s had again come close enough together to appear to justify drawing policy parallels and lessons. Some of the main economic and social problems – specifically, the loss of tax base in large cities dependent upon manufacturing industry – also appeared to be evolving in similar ways. However, in their attempts to do so, both then and subsequently, participants in the process were were apt to overlook or gloss over some of the basic differences between the two situations, which make drawing such parallels (seductive though they may seem) a perilous enterprise, and also raise other questions about whether an exclusively Anglo-American focus may not be seriously deficient, at least seen from a British point of view.

Differences in the structure of government, different expectations of the role of business and cultural differences – for example, perceptions of the role of the state towards the individual and the legitimacy of different forms of intervention and differences in population composition – are all obvious examples of these distinctions (Hambleton, 1990). Neverthelesss, they did not inhibit the use of such comparisons throughout the course of the next phase in the evolution of urban policy in the two countries.

ENTER THE NEW RIGHT

At the end of 1970s, Britain elected a government with a political agenda radically different from all its post-war predecessors (Kavanagh, 1987; Young, 1990). This agenda, with its central emphasis on the importance of reinstating individual enterprise as a motive force, with a greatly enhanced part for the private sector and a linked aspiration to 'roll back the frontiers of the state', was also substantially that of the Reagan administration elected in the following year in the United States. In both cases, these broad objectives were reflected in the approach adopted towards urban policy, perhaps best captured in the term 'privatism'. Politically, according to Sam Bass Warner, this consists of the belief that 'the community should keep the peace among individual money-makers and, if possible, help to create an open and thriving setting where each citizen should have some substantial opportunity to flourish' (quoted in Barnekov *et al.*, 1989).

These common objectives led speedily to another round of active exchanges of ideas and experience. In particular, the UK Government's concern to reanimate the role of the private sector led to the holding, in 1980, of a major Anglo-American conference at the Civil Service College, Sunningdale, under the chairmanship of the then Minister of Local government, Tom King (Boyle, 1983; Heseltine, 1986). This led in turn in the following year to the formation in Britain of 'Business in the Community', a group of senior industrialists whose objective was to promote and support 'corporate social responsibility'. This phrase, which was at that stage still comparatively seldom heard in the United Kingdom, had been a fundamental element in the private sector's approach to urban policy in the United States. The success of this first gathering led on to a series of less formal exchanges that continued throughout the 1980s, as new policies took shape on both sides of the Atlantic.

Some convergence of policy was in any case likely, regardless of the ideological preconceptions of the two administrations, in the light of the common developments already referred to above (Hambleton, 1990). Attempts were made during the 1980s by British municipal authorities, either alone or in partnership (and often in direct competition with one another) to address these problems and summon up support for strengthening their local economic base, by attracting investment from public and private sources and winning a share in new initiatives – particularly in the high-technology sector. But these were undertaken against the background of increasing fiscal pressures: a decline in the tax base, often accentuated by the withdrawal of financial support from public funds, in the British case through increasingly stringent central controls on local authority expenditure and drastic cuts in resources allocated to regional policies. In this respect, the impact of central government policy took a very similar form.

However, in other respects the response of central (national or federal) government towards these developments evolved very differently in the two countries. Although resources on a substantial scale continued to be devoted to urban policy from public sources on both sides of the Atlantic, the policy stance of the two governments was very different.

POLICY THEMES FOR THE 1980s

As already suggested, the main common theme in policy as it evolved over the 1980s in the UK and US was privatism (not to be confused with privatisation, which in this context implies entrusting the private sector with responsibility for the delivery of specific municipal services). The emphasis on privatism marched with that of partnership, which in both cases was a theme inherited by the new administrations from their predecessors. But partnership required a new definition to convey the full implications of these new departures in policy.

In Britain, deeply engrained suspicions – both in Whitehall and in most town halls – about admitting the business sector (however corporately responsible) into full association with the devising and execution of public policy had to be overturned. The Thatcher government chose to use its perception of the American experience as one lever for doing so. This process took place in a series of stages.

Michael Heseltine, as minister principally responsible at the beginning of the new government's term of office, chose initially to work within the shell of his predecessor's public sector based partnership policies, although he was subsequently sharply critical of them, commenting that they were 'a classic example of just throwing more public money at a problem without any attempt to address the problem itself' (Heseltine, 1987:138). His first step in the process of modifying these policies was the decision to turn over responsibility for two major enterprises already in hand – the regeneration of the docklands areas of London and Liverpool – to Urban Development Corporations (UDCs) modelled on the new town development corporations. These were to be single-function regeneration agencies with a brief to attract private resources through 'leverage': the use of public money to promote private investment. Second, after the race riots in several major cities (Scarman, 1981), Heseltine took responsibility for action in one of them (Liverpool). From this flowed the Merseyside Task Force, an attempt to involve the private sector directly in urban regeneration, initially through a face-to-face confrontation, promoted by Heseltine himself, involving a number of directors and senior managers of businesses with local interests (Heseltine, 1987; Parkinson and Duffy, 1984). This in turn produced the Financial Institutions Group (FIG), which provided for secondment into Whitehall of financial specialists from the private sector – a device of a kind perfectly familiar in the United States but not previously attempted on any scale in Britain (Hennessy, 1990).

The introduction of individuals from outside government ran alongside the adoption of new measures from the same source: information systems (in which Heseltine was also a ministerial pioneer) and the Financial Management Initiative (FMI), intended to introduce market disciplines into public sector management. This process, although intended to achieve changes in the culture of government at a general level, had particular relevance for the area of urban policy, where the private sector was traditionally suspicious of both the attitudes and competence of its opposite numbers in central and local government (see Mobbs, 1986).

Alongside this process of involving the private sector ran a continuing emphasis on containing and controlling the role of local authorities. The Conservative Government kept up a flow of legislation at a steady rate of one bill per year throughout most of the 1980s, all intended to limit the powers of local authorities, in respect of either the scale or scope of their expenditure. Urban local authorities – mostly under Labour control – fought back. They had their own agenda for economic regeneration, constructed on a very different basis from that of the Secretary of State. So long as their general powers were still available, local authorities used them to promote public sector led local economic policies, designed to protect existing jobs and generate new ones through devices like the creation of Local Enterprise Boards.

It was accordingly essential for the Conservative Government's strategy to be able to devise means of channelling resources into the inner-city areas in ways which would reach private sector investors, without unacceptable restrictions being imposed by local government. One such device was the creation of urban task forces – small teams of civil servants and secondees reporting direct to ministers. These were introduced into areas of high deprivation with a brief to stimulate local action, with an emphasis on job creation and the promotion of small businesses, with a particular stress, in certain cases, on the needs of ethnic minorities. The other device was one already employed in the US to draw in private sector development: the Urban Development Action Grant (UDAG).

UDAG was in fact one of the Carter administration's initiatives, inherited by Reagan. As he moved into the White House, Reagan also received the report of a Commission established by his predecessor – the McGill Commission (Barnekov et al., 1989). This advocated a further shift in policy, away from 'place' to 'people'-based programmes. Arguing that the industrial city was becoming an anachronism, the Commission's report commented that 'the best national urban strategy is the restoration of steady growth in the economy'. No centrally administered national urban policy was necessary. Instead, a locationally neutral approach favouring more private sector investment should be adopted.

It was on this foundation that the Reagan administration constructed its own policy, outlined in the President's *National Urban Policy Report* published in 1982. This set out to encourage urban adaptation to economic change, stimulate self-reliance in the cities and support urban leadership, particularly from among the business community. A key means of achieving this would be the establishment of public-private sector partnerships. A 'Presidential Task Force on Private Sector Initiatives' was established with the job of cataloguing 'ways in which private organisations, commercial, industrial and neighbourhood can, if not replace the public sector, then at least assist in the process of reducing public expenditure on, and involvement with urban affairs' (Boyle, 1983:9–10). Among the devices identified by the administration as a way of attracting the private sector into partnership was one derived from the British experience: the creation of Enterprise Zones (EZs).

Thus two techniques for achieving urban regeneration crossed the Atlantic in the early 1980s, one in each direction (UDAG and EZs). Their respective records in terms of the declared objectives of policy – principally, the promotion of investment in local economies – are instructive. Almost equally significant, however, has been the achievement of these and other parallel initiatives in terms of job creation, since it is on assertions about the capacity of these programmes to generate employment for local residents that the argument for the 'trickledown' of benefit to deprived areas and their inhabitants (especially minority groups) ultimately rests.

TWO POLICIES IN ACTION

UDAG/UDG

The Urban Development Action Grant was devised to stimulate private investment in severely distressed urban areas by supplying a capital subsidy for economic development projects, where there was a firm commitment of public resources. Its key distinguishing feature was the direct involvement of the private sector – especially its requirement that there should be a legally binding private commitment to invest in a specific project. As Barnekov comments, 'this meant that business people were brought directly and publicly into the design of a development project' (Barnekov *et al.*, 1989:73). Initially, UDAG enjoyed bipartisan support in the United States (it had been the only element in the Carter programme to be implemented without difficulties in Congress); and, by the time the wave of British visitors anxious for models for successful policy initiatives involving the private sector arrived, it had apparently successfully bedded down.

As an established American programme, UDAG was taken up by the Financial Institutions Group (FIG) that Heseltine had set up within the DoE; one of the private sector secondees, Howard Mallinson, subsequently spoke enthusiastically about the opportunities UDAG seemed to present (Hennessy, 1990:710). It became, according to Heseltine, the 'most fruitful and far reaching' of the group's proposals – and their endorsement of its practicality in the British context was decisive (Heseltine, 1987:146–7). Under the barely different title, Urban Development Grant (UDG), it was duly passed into British law. In implementing it, Regional DoE offices were instructed to look to local chambers of commerce and the business sector generally, as part of the grant assessment process (Heseltine, 1987:146). A substantial element of the DoE's urban block allocation was allocated to sustaining this programme.

However, by the mid-1980s, UDAG was in trouble in its country of origin. Expenditure on locally based schemes conflicted with the US administration's strategy of cutting direct federal expenditure on specific urban policies. The President had already made one attempt to cut the programme back, shortly after entering office. Subsequently, Reagan's Director of Budget, David Stockman, commented that 'if there was a single program . . . we inherited that was both a statist abomination and something a Republican Administration had a chance to kill outright, it was the Urban Development Action Grant program. It was called UDAG – a sincere-sounding acronym that covered a multitude of sins. PORK would have been more accurate' (Barnekov *et al.*, 1989:112). The administration's 1986 budget proposals again targeted the programme for abolition; and it barely survived to end of Reagan's second term, with a much-reduced budget.

Meanwhile, the 'statist abomination' in its British incarnation also began to provoke some second thoughts. Heseltine's enthusiasm was unabated. But an evaluation by the National Audit Office (NAO) was critical of the standards of evaluation in the first three years of the programme (1982–5), and specifically of some apparent breaches in the criteria for approving grant 'when a particularly large or prestigious project was under consideration'. Particular attention was drawn to high-profile schemes in Birmingham and Gateshead which produced private-public investment ratios of over 20: 1, raising doubts about whether any contribution from the public sector had been necessary before the schemes could proceed (NAO, 1990). Tighter financial controls were accordingly introduced; as Heseltine ruefully commented, 'the Treasury never sleeps. The UDG scheme took a battering and some flexibility has been lost' (1987:147).

But these criticisms appear relatively mild alongside the American evaluation of UDAG, which was conducted by the Center for Community Change (1988). In summary, the Center's report concluded that in one of the most important areas of potential impact, the creation of new jobs, 'developer promises of job creation are seldom matched by performance. Reporting is clouded by confusion, omissions and uncertainty. Government monitoring is passive and superficial. Meaningful evaluation is elusive'(1988:9). Mainly, this was because 'some local governments have failed . . . to ensure that developers and employers who benefit from these public subsidies live up to their commitments' (1988:45).

In short, neither in respect of the attraction of genuinely new investment nor in generation of jobs were UDG/UDAG's claims matched by performance, on either side of the Atlantic. In both countries, it has since disappeared – to be replaced in Britain by City Grant, as part of a new range of policy initiatives.

Enterprise Zones

The paternity of the Enterprise Zones concept is in some dispute: responsibility is shared between the British urban geographer Peter Hall and the former Conservative Chancellor, Sir Geoffrey Howe, who used the occasion of a speech on the Isle of Dogs in 1978 to launch a set of proposals for the promotion of enterprise by removing certain specific taxation, rating and other financial restrictions and speeding up all the relevant planning processes.

After the Conservatives came to power, eleven such zones were established, each intended to last for a 10-year period (Department of the Environment, 1981). Undertakings were given that a speedier and simpler planning regime would be enforced throughout the areas identified.

Shortly after the proposal had been implemented in Britain, a series of attempts were made to initiate similar schemes in the United States. The terms in which the case was framed were sometimes excessively hyperbolic: for example, Meir and Gelzer (1982) introduced their discussion by commenting that 'from time to time there emerges an issue, such as war, or an idea, such as placing a man on the moon, that fires the frontier spirit and forges a broad political coalition'. Enterprise Zones (EZs) became one of the few distinctive new proposals among Reagan's urban policies. But the results achieved bore little relationship to the rhetoric.

Although federal proposals for introduction of enterprise zones failed to get through Congress, 32 states adopted some form of zone programme – producing 1400 individual schemes in all. Subsequent evaluations in the United States failed to uncover any clinching evidence of the effectiveness of such zones, citing instead their psychological value as statements chiming in with the notion of 'getting government off business's back'. Deregulation has not proved to be a significant factor in attracting new investment; and 'tax holidays' have only a temporary effect (often at the expense of adjoining areas with similar needs').

The Center for Community Change evaluation (1988) was once again particularly dismissive, citing the Director of Hartford's Development Commission as observing that 'the Enterprise Zone is a sham. All talk. It is a public relations ploy without meaningful subsidies. What subsidies do exist are ones that do not enable firms to do anything they couldn't already do with existing State programs' (1988:37). All in all, an ironic reversal of Halsey's theory – the revolutionary innovation proving 'soggy on arrival' from the UK.

In Britain, the story has been much the same, with one striking exception. The NAO reported on progress with Zones in 1988, to the effect that the evidence was inclusive and the case required further examination if some pressing anxieties were to be satisfied. The DoE commissioned consultants who found in 1987 that in total, at a cost to public funds of just under £300 million, the eleven Enterprise Zones had generated between them 10,500 new permanent jobs (after allowing for displacement). The net cost of creating each new job was therefore £30,000. In December 1987, the Secretary of State (having presumably done his arithmetic) announced that there would be no general extension of the EZ scheme.

The spectacular exception to the rule that EZs have made only a marginal impact was the case of the Isle of Dogs, which had been the place where the whole notion of creating zones had first been floated. As a result of a series of developments that were not anticipated – by either the government, the Docklands Development Corporation or indeed the private sector – the Isle of Dogs became the focus of a gigantic office-led construction boom stimulated by the rapidly growing needs of the City of London for new accommodation in anticipation of the 'big bang' – the deregulation of financial services. The concessions offered on the Isle of Dogs through the EZ played a significant part in attracting this investment in new construction, which led in turn to rents and land values rising dramatically inside the EZ (47 per cent higher, according to the 1987 report). As the first chairman of the London Docklands Development Corporation (LDDC) put it, 'it's not a brilliant record in creating jobs . . . but it's a pretty good record in filling up the Isle of Dogs, which is our first priority' (Brownill, 1990). Whether what filled the Isle of Dogs is a socially, aesthetically or even economically desirable outcome is another story.

Thus Enterprise Zones, like UDG/UDAG, failed to match promise with performance; but the Isle of Dogs episode did help to point the direction of the next phase of urban policy in Britain.

PRIVATISM IN FULL FLOWER: THEN GONE TO SEED?

British urban policy entered a new phase after the third successive Conservative victory at the General Election of June 1987 and the Prime Minister's election night promise to do something about 'those inner cities'. The obvious direction in which to move appeared to be that already identified in the London Docklands – the leveraging in of private sector funds, especially from the property sector, riding giddily upwards on the back of the boom in values of the late 1980s in the south-east. This was the approach already signalled by the then Minister for Housing, Urban Affairs and Construction, John Patten, in a *Guardian* article shortly before the election. 'The public-sector dominated municipal solutions of the past simply have not worked,' he asserted. 'They have made things worse because they were based on a misunderstanding of what makes cities – and other areas – successful. We should draw a line under them' (Patten, 1987).

Instead, Patten proposed an expansion of the approach based on Urban Development Corporations, so 'spectacularly' successful in London Docklands. 'Cities grew and flourished', he concluded, 'because of private enterprise and municipal pride; it is private enterprise, backed by helpful, direct and concentrated government action that will renew them'. Concentration, in this concept, would take the form of the creation of a new group of UDCs, some in areas of dereliction without substantial resident populations, but others imposed on major cities (Leeds, Manchester, Cardiff,

Bristol, Sheffield) and all without benefit of consent from the local authorities representing the areas chosen.

But even the establishment of further UDCs would hardly by itself match the scale of the then Prime Minister's aspirations for a fundamental economic (and political) transformation. The government's newly designated coordinator of inner-city programmes, Kenneth Clarke, was accordingly despatched on the now traditional whistle-stop tour of the United States in search of fresh ideas.

It was crucial to the success of the new approach to secure an enhanced commitment by the private sector to underwriting the success of new policy initiatives – for example, by strengthening the identification between private corporations and their 'home towns' – which had appeared to be a particularly significant factor in the United States. As a first step in this process, the role of Business in the Community (BiC) and their work in promoting local enterprise agencies were to be promoted through moves to bind them more closely into the government's programmes. The individual entrusted with this responsibility was Sir Hector Laing, Chairman of United Biscuits; the effort was diversified by the creation of the Per Cent Club operating under the patronage of Prince Charles, members of which pledged to give not less than 0.5 per cent of profits to community training programmes. Sir Hector himself told the AGM of the BiC in 1987 that: 'the major public challenge of today is the regeneration of our deprived urban areas. The PM has declared the government's intention to mount a campaign to meet this challenge and has called on the private sector for support and cooperation. We must respond – and I am calling on you, the private sector – to support a comprehensive package of long term programmes to address the problems of the inner cities' (*Guardian*, 6 January 1988).

On his return from the US, Clarke's main energies were put into promoting the commitment of the private sector across the country (his so-called 'breakfast shows'), promoting the notion that: 'businessmen in the past provided the leadership that made their cities great. The city fathers, heroes of mine such as Joseph Chamberlain, combined political leadership with business leadership and made their cities what they became a century or so ago. That can be done again in modern circumstances' (Clarke, 1988b).

The terms of the deal being struck with the private sector became evident on the publication in March 1988 of the government's plans, *Action for Cities* (HMSO, 1988), essentially a glossy compendium of existing government policies larded with flattering references to the private sector but pointedly overlooking both the functions and the achievements of local authorities. This approach was underpinned by stressing the role of UDCs as vehicles for urban regeneration and of inner-city task forces as locally based brokers between the public and private sectors. The proposed partnership between 'business and enterprise' and central government, to the exclusion of local authorities, was also consistent with both the government's general policies towards local government *and* the specific proposals being promoted by Nicholas Ridley for the progressive removal of local authorities from their role in service delivery (Ridley, 1988).

The clinching of the private sector's commitment was provided by the Confederation of British Industry, which set up a Task Force at its annual conference in 1987 to produce guidelines for future private sector involvement in urban regeneration. These were published in the following September as *Initiatives Beyond Charity* (CBI, 1988). The report places particular emphasis on the importance of assembling high-profile groups of local community business leaders to 'provide the vision and leadership necessary to mobilise local business resources'. Such vision 'needs to be both bold and practical', identifying 'flagship' projects that will project the image of the city as a place for new investment. The CBI Task Force explicitly based their approach on their perception of what had been successfully undertaken in the United States – Baltimore is cited as the key example, complete with statutory colour photograph. Certainly, there were aspects of the Baltimore experience which did seem to lend themselves particularly to imitation: a high-profile development scheme; a responsible – and responsive – local business sector; an executive mayor capable of delivering practical support and a positive profile from the public sector side.

On the basis of this perception, the CBI team and the government have encouraged similar initiatives – notably in Glasgow and in Newcastle, in which the City fathers, as the local business leadership are (quite unhistorically) taken to be, have been encouraged to play a facilitating role. However, in the course of this process and as part of the parallel developments in cities in which the second and third generation UDCs were introduced, a number of difficulties have arisen.

These centre mainly on the role of local government. It rapidly became apparent that the initial *Action for Cities* technique of simply ignoring local government simply wouldn't answer. Local government's capacities had changed over the course of the 1980s as they became more closely involved in the processes of economic development and learnt some of the skills and imperatives which entering that field imposed. Attitudes, too, shifted as authorities became both better informed and more constructive in their approach to the private sector. The new public sector management culture spread to local government and took root. Evidence began to emerge – notably in Scotland, where different structures and a more cooperative environment made collaboration easier – of apparently successful experiments in partnership between public and private sectors; for example, the GEAR experiment in the East End of Glasgow (Donnison and Middleton, 1987).

Moreover, central government's attitudes towards local authorities came in for severe criticism in an important report produced by the Audit Commission (1989). Recognising the importance of the change of attitude on the part of local government, the Commission called for 'a greater consistency of approach and coordination by central government [and] a willingness to recognise the appropriate role of local authorities. Their ability to respond to local circumstances should not be unreasonably constrained' (1989:2). Visiting American observers drew the same conclusion, this time on the basis of the American experience. Peter Henschel, a former deputy mayor of San Francisco seconded to work with Business in the Community, commented that he was 'shocked at central government attitudes towards local authorities', who they were treating 'as though they were adolescents not to be trusted with the family car' (Henschel, 1989).

One of the consequences of this attitude, as Henschel pointed out, was neglect of the social dimension of inner-city regeneration, 'often the last thing thought about'. He added: 'the worst example in Britain is undoubtedly the London Docklands development' (Henschel, 1989). This was a conclusion also reached by a number of other critics, notably the House of Commons Employment Committee, which had produced a scathing report on the failure of the Docklands Development Corporation to sustain an adequate training programme or to secure jobs for local people (1988). This was only one item among the accumulating evidence that private sector led urban regeneration spread benefits very unevenly; and that the theory that national economic growth would take care of the problems of the disadvantaged in the inner city by a process of 'trickle down' was seriously deficient (ESRC, 1985). Claims in successive UK government documents to that effect were not backed by any substantial evidence (in practice, they could cite only the general fall in unemployment, which lasted until mid-1990 and then rapidly reversed itself). On the question of the Docklands, whose 'flagship' status made ministers and civil servants especially sensitive, the response to criticism in successive inquiries (House of Commons, 1988; National Audit Office, 1988, 1990; London Docklands Consultative Committee, 1990) was to the effect that opportunities for physical redevelopment had to be seized when they presented themselves and that benefits for locals (especially jobs) could be sought as a spin-off from development by direct negotiation with developers. But in practice, as the inquiries showed, these benefits failed to materialise on any substantial scale.

This lesson could in fact have been learned by any visitor to the United States prepared to venture beyond the standard whistle-stops and take in some of the deprived neighbourhoods outside the immediate city centre

(Ward, 1989; Hambleton, 1990). Even the much cited case of Baltimore displays the same characteristics. As Barnekov and his colleagues demonstrate (1989: 94–5), 'indicators of the aggregate economic health of Baltimore continue to reflect stagnation or actual decline rather than a thriving city, successfully adapting to economic change' and 'despite the downtown investment and signs of restoration around the waterfront, Baltimore's public-private partnership resulted in limited and uneven development'. They add: 'Baltimore's redevelopment program has not benefited the majority of city dwellers and its overall economic performance has not matched that of other comparable cities. Despite these shortcomings, Baltimore has achieved undisputed success in image management' (1989:94–5).

In short, Baltimore was not after all (despite the CBI's advocacy) the ideal model for Britain's Glasgows and Newcastles to follow. Nor at national level was the progressive withdrawal of direct reponsibility for urban policy by the US federal government over the course of the 1980s – which has contrasted so sharply with the hyperactivity of the central state in the UK. Although attempts have been made to generate an alternative agenda in some American cities – especially those cities that have elected black and minority group politicians to executive positions (Judd and Ready, 1986) – the viability of the US as a role model had declined sharply by the end of the Reagan presidency.

Indeed, by 1990, the whole notion of the private sector based partnerships generating solutions ceased to command much credibility. The Barnekov team's analysis concludes (1989:225) that 'in both the US and Britain, advocates of privatism as a strategy of urban regeneration have exaggerated its benefits and largely ignored its costs'. Partly, there was always a substantial element of dishonesty about the claims made on behalf of this approach. A substantial underpinning of public funds was always an indispensable ingredient, even at the peak of achievement. Michael Parkinson (1987), reviewing the Boston experience, was told by a local banker to 'tell Mrs Thatcher there isn't a single piece of urban renewal which would have gone ahead in this country without huge sums of public money'.

Even at the height of its apparent success, when 'leverage' rates of 10 or 12: 1 in private sector investment were being claimed, LDDC was still consuming a disproportionate share of the DoE's urban block budget. When the recession came and property values in London were particularly hard hit, the Development Corporation was in the middle of a belated attempt to devise a social programme and make good the deficiencies in infrastructure (especially transportation) blithely ignored in the years of rapid expansion. Its only answer in this predicament was to make a further call on public funds – which seem unlikely to be sufficient to rescue the social programmes. But these, in turn, are the only substantial hope of tangible benefit for local inhabitants, given the failure of the Development Corporation to strike hard enough deals with developers of major schemes while the economic going was still good, despite the initial willingness of such developers, on the basis of their American experience, to accept an obligation to provide jobs for locals (see Olympia and York's evidence to the House of Commons Employment Committee, 1988 on the Canary Wharf development).

So the private sector partnership model (for the moment, at least) has lost its gloss; although how much this was a product of the recession which began to take effect in Britain in 1990 and has also affected some ambitious private sector developments in the US – those of James Rouse, for example (Hambleton, 1990) – remains to be seen. By 1992, property firms were collapsing with monotonous regularity, most conspicuously of all the Reichmann brothers' Olympia and York company, whose Canary Wharf development had been the main showpiece for Docklands regeneration. Certainly recent experience in Britain of urban regeneration based on property development has powerfully underlined the force of the proposition that in the last analysis 'you can't buck the market' – especially if the basic assumption on which your policies rest is that regeneration is a matter for the operation of market forces.

Meanwhile, another question remains: was Kenneth Clarke right in asserting that the US is the only country from which Britain can learn about partnerships as a means of addressing urban issues, or are there after all possible alternatives?

SOME LESSONS FROM THE HEXAGON?

The case histories just described do not offer much support for the proposition that policies based on the assumption that market-based approaches are intrinsically superior to state-led programmes will necessarily be more successful than those that rest on different premises. This, in turn, suggests that there might be more benefit in looking at other societies where such alternative approaches have actually been followed during the post-war period.

More specifically, in both the British model and (though to a lesser extent) the American, partnership between private and public sectors is conducted on the premise that there will normally be conflicts of interests – based on a divergence of cultures – between the two partners, even if these may be temporarily suspended in pursuit of particular policy goals. There are other models, however, of which the French is perhaps the most interesting.

As suggested at the outset, the British tendency to look exclusively at Anglophone countries for policy lessons is normally validated by reference to cultural differences between Britain and other European countries; and by perceived structural and functional variations between systems of government across (and beyond) the European Community. There is some – though not all that much – truth in these objections; but they have demonstrably not prevented helpful comparisons being drawn (see Stewart and Clarke, 1990).

The French case is potentially of particular interest because that society passed through a comparatively rapid process of modernisation in the course of the 1960s which has led in turn to an extended period of sustained economic growth. This period of expansion was characterised by a deliberate attempt to spread the benefits of growth outside the capital by creating so-called *metropoles d'équilibre*, centring on major provincial cities. The resources allocated under this and other programmes have been directed in part to achieving large-scale physical regeneration of the centres of these cities (LeGales, 1991).

These two developments, taken together, have had important consequences for the urban situation in France. The country as a whole has largely escaped the deepest troughs of economic recession in the last two decades, even if it also failed to experience the dizzy peaks of growth that the British briefly enjoyed in the later 1980s. This in turn has facilitated the rapid creation of a modernised infrastructure and good-quality public services. Furthermore, with a few conspicuous exceptions, French cities have escaped the impact of the rapid contraction in manufacturing industry that has had such disastrous consequences for many British and American cities.

The fact that, for the most part, industrialisation came later in France and has tended to be concentrated away from the older centres of population has meant that social and economic problems have tended to be located elsewhere, on the periphery of major cities rather than in their centres – which have neither lost population nor experienced problems of acute dereliction and deprivation. In this sense, France can be said not to have an 'inner-city problem' as such – which is not the same as saying there are no urban problems (LeGales, 1991). At the same time, the political system has been subject to an experiment in decentralisation of political power – initiated during the first *septennat* of President Mitterrand and still in the process of implementation (Ashford, 1990).

Despite passing through this period of fundamental change, the French polity has retained certain distinctive characteristics which have helped to shape outcomes (and distinguish them from developments described earlier in this paper). These could be summarised as follows:

– continued acceptance of the legitimacy of the role of the state in social and economic policy;
– similarly, a belief that there is still a role (if an attentuated one) for a form of central planning;

- acceptance on both sides of a basic community of interest between public and private sectors, underpinned by regular exchanges of staff at senior level as part of normal career patterns;
- the existence of a number of joint public–private agencies functioning over a long period in a number of roles within the urban system; leading to
- a willingness to take pragmatic positions on the merits or drawbacks of such questions as privatisation (enshrined in President Mitterrand's 'ni–ni' proposition – that is, neither more nationalisation nor more privatisation, although this is now in the course of modification);
- a strong tradition of local government at the most basic level of all (the commune) and upwards and of the executive and representational role of its political head, the *maire*, who participates in an elaborate web of political relationships which links them into the national political structures (Mabileau *et al.*, 1987).

These conditions have permitted a number of joint agencies to operate in a number of crucial service areas – starting with water and extending to electricity, housing, transport, public works and building. At the local level, this 'semi-public' sector takes the form of SEMs (sociétés d'entreprise mixtes), which make individual deals with municipalities for the delivery of services (Digings, 1990).

Dominique Lorrain (1990), who has made an extended study of these systems of service delivery, suggests that they may have considerable relevance for the effective delivery of urban services in other countries, subject to the qualification that the form they take is determined by some specific features of the French political system. They have also adapted their operations to the new political context of the 1980s, which has seen the emergence of a more active political role for urban *maires*, who have taken on the explicit function of developing local economic policy. The *maires'* role as entrepreneurs acting as mediators between local public and private sectors and mobilising resources from higher up the system – using the network of the *notables* with its connexions up to the top – is captured in the characteristic press image of the municipal 'locomotive'.

In managerial terms, this role is increasingly discharged through appointing deputy mayors as managers, with specific responsibility for such joint initiatives. This forms part of a wider process of professionalising French local government, a process accelerated by the transfer downwards of a significant number of powers under the decentralisation programme and the impact of the introduction of new managerial techniques and attitudes (Sorbets, 1989).

The key to the French approach is the retention of political legitimacy, which is 'above technical legitimacy and restrains professionalism' (Lorrain,

1990). This is not the case in the Anglo-Saxon systems, where political leadership has played a more limited role at local level in the partnerships that have emerged in the course of the 1980s. The persistence of adversarial politics in UK local government is also regarded by the private sector as a positive obstacle to the implementation of new initiatives for urban regeneration (see Mobbs, 1986). In France, by contrast, partnership is institutionalised and the partners can coexist comfortably within the political system. As Hoffmann-Martinot summarises it (1989:18):

> The municipal experience between 1983 and 1989, the ideological shifts currently taking place (the decline of the left-right cleavage) and the growing professionalisation of municipal employees (more and more conscious of the need to modernise services) are all factors likely to encourage in the coming years the search for innovatory and pragmatic developments in local public management. In these circumstances, one cannot help wishing partnership a long life.

All this is not to say that instant transplantation is possible – or, indeed, that the French do not have their share of acute urban problems, especially in satellite HLM ('*habitations à loyers modérés*') estates with substantial immigrant populations. The institution in 1982 of a National Commission with responsibility for promoting social development in the *quartiers* and the programme of action that followed, taking in 400 different areas, with substantial investment in community facilities did not prevent outbreaks of violence taking place. These broke out in 1990 at Vaulx-en-Velan on the outskirts of Lyons and in 1991 in Mantes-la-Jolie in the Seine valley, which possesses by far the largest high-rise housing estate in France. Nevertheless, the dramatic improvement in the general level of public service delivery over the post-war period suggests that the French alternative may be worth serious consideration as an alternative model for partnership.

SOME CONCLUSIONS

Have partnerships based on privatism failed, as Barnekov and his collaborators confidently assert? If so, is this because they are basically flawed, or as an unforeseen consequence of other developments (economic recession coming at an unfortunate time, at least for UK policies)? Or is it because they have failed to deliver the promised substantial benefits to the populations of the urban areas within which the experiments of the 1980s have been conducted (cf. *Action for Cities*)?

To ask these questions is to raise some basic issues about the objectives of urban regeneration policies. There is a sense in which to make judgements about the immediate local consequences of policy is to be guilty of naivete about their real objectives. Certainly, the goals of the partnership policies were framed in terms of the mutual benefits that would accrue to investors and resident populations, with central government as *tertium gaudens*; but the flimsiness of the evidence for any substantial gains by the ostensible 'partners' in the local community suggests that other undeclared objectives might also have been on the agenda.

One way of exploring what the basic objectives of policy have been during the past decade may be to establish who really benefits from them, in practice. Who gains from urban restructuring? Is it a reorganisation of urban space to fit the imperatives of post-Fordist modes of production, as Paul Hoggett (1987) argues? Is it about political control of the urban system – making sure that minority ethnic groups can never enjoy full access to all the potential benefits of the urban economy? Is it about social control – the law and order agenda – or simply avoiding another repetition of urban rioting? Such is the impression left by recent attempts to subsume the issue of inner city policies in another debate, on the alleged urban 'underclass', whose irredeemable failings are held by some American social scientists to make the task of urban regeneration impossible (Murray, 1990). Or is it simply about efficient management, applying depoliticised technocracy, which also – almost, but not quite, coincidentally – offers the best prospects for making profits?

Alternatively, there is the possibility of pursuing another agenda, which is about empowerment. This agenda is concerned with participation and the creation of 'transparent' systems of government, with clear points of access. This has by definition (almost) to be a system of local governance – although there is an alternative consumerist model of empowerment. Arguably, it is the empowerment-as-citizen approach which best serves to bring back the social agenda that has been lost in the private-partnership approach, in which the rising tide sinks some of the boats instead of lifting them all, as its protagonists like to maintain (Deakin and Wright, 1990).

If this alternative is to be given serious consideration, it must begin with the acknowledgement that in the UK, at least, local government in the past has been unable to deliver, either singly or in those partnerships in which it has so far been involved. However, there is a new momentum behind the current trends towards autonomy and self-management – the decentralisation *and* quality movement (Gaster, 1991) – which suggests that, instead of sawing off the local government branch, as central government in UK has been busy doing for the last 15 years, it might be worth trying to use it to implement a new form of partnership involving public and private sectors with people in the locality, on terms that don't exclude the social agenda.

REFERENCES

Anglo-American Conference on Experiments in Social Policy (1969) Ditchley Park, Oxfordshire, 29–31 October, mimeo.

Ashford, D. (1990) 'Decentralising France: how the socialists discovered pluralism', *West European Politics* 13(4).

Audit Commission (1989) *Urban Regeneration and Economic Development: the Local Government Dimension*, London: HMSO.

Barnekov, T., Boyle, R. and Rich, D. (1989) *Privatism and Urban Policy in Britain and the United States*, Oxford: Oxford University Press.

Boyle, R. (1983) *Privatising Urban Problems: A commentary on Anglo-American Urban Policy*, Glasgow: Centre for the Study of Public Policy.

Brownill, S. (1990) *Developing London's Docklands*, London: Paul Chapman.

Center for Community Change (1988) 'Bright promises, questionable results', mimeo.

Clarke, Kenneth (1988a) . . . 'hits road to Inner City renewal', *The Independent*, 4 January.

—— (1988b) 'Private cash targetted to fund plans for cities', *The Independent*, 8 March.

Community Development Projects (1977a) *The Costs of Industrial Change*, London: CDP Inter-Project Team.

—— (1977b) *Gilding the Ghetto*, London: CDP Inter-Project Team.

Confederation of British Industry (1988) *Initiatives beyond Charity*, London: CBI.

Deakin, N. and Wright, A.W. (eds) (1990) *Consuming Public Services*, London: Routledge.

Department of the Environment (1981) *Enterprise Zones*, London: HMSO.

Digings, L. (1990) *Competitive Tendering and the European Communities*, London: Association of London Authorities.

Donnison, D.V. and Middleton, A. (eds) (1987) *Regenerating the Inner City, Glasgow's Experience*, London: Routledge.

ESRC Research Team (1985) *Changing Cities*, London: ESRC.

Gaster, L. (1991) *Quality at the Front Line*, Bristol: School for Advanced Urban Studies.

Hambleton, R. (1990) *Urban government in the 1990s; Lessons from the USA*, Bristol: School for Advanced Urban Studies.

—— (1991) 'The regeneration of US and British cities', *Local Government Studies* (5), September/October, 53–69.

Hennessy, P. (1990) *Whitehall*, London: Fontana Books.

Henschel, P. (1989) 'Public and private partnership in urban regeneration', *Royal Institute of Public Administration Report*, Winter, 5–6.

HMSO (1977) *Policy for the Inner Cities*, London.

—— (1988) *Action for Cities*, London.

Heseltine, M. (1987) *Where there's a Will*, London: Hutchinson.

Higgins, J., Deakin, N., Edwards, J. and Wicks, M. (1983) *Government and Urban Poverty*, Oxford: Blackwell.

Hoggett, P. (1987) 'A farewell to mass production?' in P. Hoggett and R. Hambleton, *Decentralisation and Democracy*, Bristol: School for Advanced Urban Studies.

Hoffmann-Martinot, Vincent (1989) 'Concurrence et performances dans les services publics locaux: objectifs, principes et modalités d'applications', mimeo.

House of Commons Employment Committee (1988) *The Employment Effect of UDCs*, HC 327–1, London: HMSO.

Judd, D.R. and Ready, R.L. (1986) 'Entrepreneurial cities and the new politics of economic development' in G. Peterson and C.W. Lewis (eds) *Reagan and the Cities*, Washington: Urban Institute Press.

Kavanagh, D. (1987) *Thatcherism and the Decline of Consensus*, Oxford: Oxford University Press.

LeGales, Patricke (1991) 'Those French inner cities? Comparative comments on the urban crisis in Britain and France' in Michael Keith and Alisdair Rogers (eds) *Hollow Promises? Rhetoric and Reality in the Inner City*, London: Mansell.

London Docklands Consultative Committee (1990) *The Docklands Experiment*, London: LDCC.

Loney, M. (1983) *Community Against Government* London: Heinemann.

Lorrain, D. (1990) 'Public goods and private operators in France' in Richard Batley and Gerry Stoker (eds) *Local Government in Europe*, London: Macmillan.

Mabileau, A., Moyser, G., Parry, G. and Quantin, P. (1987) *Les Citoyens et la politique locale*, Paris: Pedone.

Marris, P. (1982) *Community Planning and Conceptions of Change*, London: Routledge & Kegan Paul.

Meir R. and Gelzer, S.E. (1982) 'State Enterprise Zones: the new frontier', *Urban Affairs Quarterly* 18(1).

Mobbs, N. (1986) *The Inner Urban Challenge*, London: Aims of Industry.

Murray, C. (1990) *The Emerging British Underclass*, London: Institute for Economic Affairs.

National Audit Office (1988) *Report on Department of Environment programmes*, London: HMSO.

—— (1990) *Regenerating the Inner City*, HC169, London: HMSO.

Parkinson, M. (1987) 'American cities', *New Society*, 9 October 1987.

Parkinson, M. and Duffy, J. (1984) 'The Minister for Merseyside and the Task Force', *Parliamentary Affairs* 37(1), Winter 76–96.

Patten, J. (1987) 'Inner city Big Bang', *Guardian*, 17 April.

Ridley, N. (1988) *The Enabling Local Authority*, London: Centre for Policy Studies.

Rose, R. (ed.) (1974) *Lessons from America*, London: Macmillan.

Scarman, Lord (1981) *Report on Inner City Disturbances*, London: HMSO.

Sorbets, C. (1989) 'Services urbains et gestion locale: translocal express' in C. Lalu (ed.) *Services urbains et gestion locale*, Paris: Ministre de l'Urbanisme, du Logement et des Transports.

Stewart, J.D. and Clarke, M. (1990) 'The future of local government: some lessons from Europe', mimeo.

Ward, C. (1989) *Welcome, Thinner City*, London: Bedford Square Press.

Young, H. (1990) *One of Us*, London: Fontana.

6 Returner and retainer policies for women

Short-term or long-term gains?

Jaqi Nixon and Valerie Williamson

INTRODUCTION

In 1990 the Working Mothers' Association in Britain announced: 'this is the age of the woman returner. For the first time in decades employers are turning their attentions to you' (WMA, 1990). Certainly an increasing number of British employers appeared to be taking action. A recent study in Newcastle showed that 80 per cent of local employers were taking steps to encourage women back into their employ. They were offering an increasing diversity of retainer and returner schemes and, in the words of Boots Ltd, were 'constantly coming up with fresh options, new ways to accommodate each different set of needs, circumstances and aspirations' (WMA, 1990). The *Guardian* noted too that 'Companies are offering flexible hours and better conditions to recruit and retain more women workers.' (Weston, 1990). But why were employers in Britain suddenly showing such interest in women returning to work? There appear to be a number of possible explanations.

First, employers were facing a shortage of skilled and experienced workers, partly because of a relatively buoyant market in some sectors of the economy, and partly as a consequence of a temporary reduction in the pool of available, trainable young people. (A 25 per cent reduction in the number of school leavers in the early 1990s was predicted; Rajan and Van Eupen, 1989.) The National Health Service, for example, is unable to recruit enough school leavers into nursing and yet it is estimated that, in 1992, it would have to attract more than half the 22,500 young women who leave school annually with appropriate qualifications, if a major crisis in the health service is to be averted. The government's preferred option is to attract older women into nursing (Nevill *et al.*, 1990).

Second, it is argued that women will also be required to make good the deficit in 'quality' workers, not merely in numbers. They will be needed 'at the top as well as the bottom' (Casey and McCrae, 1990). Employers, it seems, are also discovering that women make good employees and so are worth holding on to. In a study of good employer practices, for instance, Rajan and Van Eupen were able to conclude that 'in the changing world of work, women are a valuable resource in their own right, irrespective of demographic down-turn' (1989: 17). By the year 2000, it is estimated that of the 1 million more people in employment since 1988, 90 per cent will be women (*Employment Gazette*, April 1989).

Third, rising standards of living and the growth of the consumer society have made two wage-earners, rather than one breadwinner, appear a necessity (Jensen *et al.*, 1988). In addition, greater marital instability and an increase in single-parent families, further reinforced by rising educational standards of women and the influence of feminism (Chalude and Liessein-Norman, 1987), have highlighted the importance for women of economic independence. Women now feel not merely a need to work but the right to work. Thus, according to Halsall (1990), 'there is a workforce out there keen to work and waiting to offer a lot'.

Fourth, political support is also beginning to mobilise behind increased employment opportunities for women. The Labour Party Manifesto for 1987 contained a section supporting women's rights, nursery education for all 3–4 year olds and a Ministry for Women; and at a recent annual conference the party supported better access to child care for working mothers (*Guardian*, 21 September 1990). The Tory Party in government, meanwhile, has awarded tax concessions to workplace nurseries and the Department of Employment has joined with 'Woman's Hour' to launch a nationwide campaign, 'Back to the Future', to encourage women with families back to work (New Ways to Work, 1990b).

Finally, it could be argued that both government and employers, recognising the sharper competitive edge that post-1992 will supply in respect of worker recruitment, and conscious that Britain, generally, is regarded as a 'laggard' on most indicators of women's employment, are anxious to catch up with their European partners.

It may be that returner policies are of especial importance in Britain because of the relatively higher proportion of British women who remain out of paid work for the duration of their period of child-rearing. In France, for instance, the proportion of mothers who remain in work through child-rearing is 31.6 per cent compared with 3.4 per cent in Britain (Dex and Walters in McCrae, 1990). Even in families with three children the proportion of mothers remaining in work is as high as 15.5 per cent compared with 1.1 per cent for British mothers. Thus the problems associated with long spells away from paid employment, such as lack of up-to-date skills and knowledge, and lack of self-confidence, may well be more acute for women in Britain whose absence from paid work is likely to be greater.

While they might appear to meet the needs of British women however, returner programmes require close scrutiny since they are potentially exploitative. They often include the offer of part-time work, which is traditionally associated with low-status jobs and unsocial hours, attracts poor conditions of employment and is insecure. If employers are now beginning to entice women into work with offers of job share, flexible arrangements and additional attractions, there will be a need to ensure that these apparent benefits do not lead ultimately into low-paid work with poor prospects.

Part-time work continues to appeal to employers in Britain, since a number of social policies tilt the balance in this direction. Dex and Walters have shown, for example, that in neither France nor America 'have [national] insurance incentives or job protection provisions developed around the criterion of hours of work', whereas in Britain there exist a number of incentives for employers to continue to provide part-time work. These include the low earnings threshold for national insurance contributions, which affects about 2.5 million workers, and the exclusion from employment protection legislation for those working less than 10 hours a week. These same policies continue to make part-time work, from the employee's point of view, insecure and unprotected work. On the other hand, and in conflict with these policies, the social security system in Britain actually discourages people from participating in more flexible forms of work because, fuelled by a concern not to undermine full-time work incentives, earnings disregards are calculated on a weekly basis rather than being spread over a longer period (McLaughlin, 1989). In addition, and for single parents in particular, lack of an earnings disregard in the tax system to cover the costs of working can make the transfer from benefits dependence to employment a hazardous affair (Brown, 1989).

Thus it is important for women wanting to return to work that welfare policies are integrated with labour market policies in such a way as to prevent either a sharp loss of benefits or high marginal tax rates constructing barriers to their employment (Sharp and Broomhill, 1988). The fact that in the UK, unlike in other OECD countries, the proportion of single parents in the labour market has actually decreased from 22 per cent in 1978–80 to 17 per cent in 1983–5 (Millar, 1989), suggests that a lack of integration between policies may be especially in evidence. Certainly, without a coherent overall strategy at central government level, that integrates the separate policy areas in such a way as to avoid confusion and contradiction, and that provides a framework for the policies and practices of individual employers, it is difficult to see how women will derive genuine long-term benefit from potentially attractive recent developments.

At present, women's experience of paid work is predicated upon employer needs, and upon how employees can use women to meet these needs, rather than by women's own requirements as individuals, as mothers and as carers. In other words, it is employer demand for part-time workers, rather than their response to the supply of part-time women workers, which is mainly responsible for the number of hours women work and the way their paid work is organised. And where work has been organised as part-time specifically to attract women employees, this generally rests on the two untested assumptions: (a) that the work is only women's work, and (b) that women want only part-time work (Elias and Purcell in Hunt, 1988; Elias in McCrae, 1990). A number of commentators have noted how the same work can be structured by organisations to create either a full-time job when men are being recruited, or a part time and lower-paid job when women workers only are being sought (e.g. Beechay in Jensen *et al.*, 1988; Beechay and Perkins, 1987). Even the best-documented examples of changes in the organisation of work away from permanent, full-time jobs to flexible patterns of employment are generally employer driven – a reaction to economic pressures and international competition, not necessarily reflecting the needs of women.

Thus, instead of providing a 'window of opportunity', current labour market gains for women may be seen as insubstantial and insecure, much more closely tied to the needs of the labour market than to those of women. As has been suggested elsewhere, 'social justice may be more important than the needs of the labour market, but it is less pressing', therefore it is more readily shelved (*Health Services Management*, 1989).

A COMPARATIVE PERSPECTIVE

Given these concerns, can comparative analysis help us to understand better the dynamics of the situation for women, and the potential for policy intervention in the interests of equal opportunity? Looking at comparable advanced capitalist economies, in particular in Western Europe, there are clearly identifiable similarities in respect of female labour force participation. Not only in Britain are the apparent improved opportunities for women workers likely to remain dependent upon employer needs and economic fortune. Lane (1989) has provided comparative evidence to suggest this continuing association elsewhere. From her study of employment flexibility in labour markets in West Germany, France and Britain during the 1970s and 1980s, she notes the various 'economic stimuli [which] lead firms to adopt certain flexible work and/or employment practices'. Similarly, (Jensen *et al.*, 1988: 68) has demonstrated how, in France, equal opportunity policies 'have developed in a context in which their effects . . . have been overwhelmed by the state's concern with reducing the unemployment rate and restructuring French industry to make it internationally competitive'. And even in Sweden, usually identified as having a very positive stance on equal opportunities both in the workplace and in the home (Moss, 1988), the economic crisis of the early 1980s has been cited as a reason for failing to make greater progress during the 1980s (Ruggie in Jensen *et al.* 1988). Finally, as Buckley and Anderson (1988: 10) remind us, even Article 119 of the Treaty of Rome, which binds states to the principle of equal pay for equal work, was not an example of the European Commission taking a lead in equal opportunity policy: 'Rather it was inspired by the desire to ensure equal competition between states'.

Of particular importance for women wanting to work have been the increasing opportunities provided by public sector welfare services. Rein, in his analysis of the social welfare industry (SWI) in four Western democracies, has noted that in Sweden, for example, almost 90 per cent of the increase in female labour participation between 1960 and 1981 was accounted for by jobs in the SWI. And by 1983 no less than 45 per cent of all employed women in Sweden worked in the SWI. In the USA, by comparison, the SWI accounted for 28 per cent and in Britain 26 per cent of jobs held by women (in Klein and O'Higgins, 1985). This suggests, therefore, that employment opportunities for many women are predicated not only upon the vagaries of the market place but also upon the extent to which governments intend to sustain or reduce their public sector, as part of an economic strategy, and the extent to which they succeed in doing so. The impact on women of Reagan's policies of reducing federal government programmes is a case in point. Brackman *et al.* have noted, for example, that an estimated 1,000,000 federal government employees and a further 700,000 state or local government workers in public human services lost their jobs in 1981–84, and that women in particular 'walked Reagan's retrenchment plank' (in Jensen *et al.*, 1988: 220). In Britain, too, important changes are under way in the public services sector, namely contracting out, internal markets and individual contracts of employment, which bring the sharp winds of the private sector into the offices and corridors of the public sector. Some commentators have suggested that these changes within the public services will have a more serious effect upon low-paid workers, a disproportionate number of whom are black and ethnic minority women (Huws *et al.*, 1989). In some countries, such as Sweden and France, the state, as employer, is traditionally seen as giving a lead in respect of improving working conditions and arrangements for women (Walters and Crompton in McCrae, 1990). Thus any diminution in the role of the state could be viewed as a retrograde step for women workers.

Thus comparative example offers further evidence that more recent improvements in policies and practices affecting women in paid work are not really to be understood as part of an evolution of employer beneficence. If recent gains are to be safeguarded for the future, it would seem appropriate to recognise their fragility and their ultimate dependence upon market forces. Moreover, they should also be seen in the context of existing inequalities, not only between men and women but also between groups of women with different domestic responsibilities and located in different segments of the labour market. Again, a comparison between Western economies only highlights just how pervasive and well entrenched these inequalities are.

The EOC reported in 1988 that a segregated workforce is an international phenomenon, with women concentrated both in a small number of industrial categories and in particular types of work. In Europe generally, women are to be found in certain occupations – secretarial, typing, nursing, midwifery, and care and cleaning work (Buckley and Anderson, 1988). In the UK such concentrations are also pronounced, despite some improvement since 1975 when sex discrimination legislation was first introduced (Millar, 1989). Women still occupy only 7 per cent of senior executive jobs and 1 per cent of managing directorships (Rajan and Van Eupen, 1989). By contrast, 25 per cent of full-time women manual workers are in packing, painting and assembly (*Labour Research*, March 1990), and the largest proportion of non-manual women workers are undertaking clerical or related work, while a large minority are employed in education, health and welfare professions (*Employment Gazette*, December 1990). Of mothers working full time, 27 per cent have been identified as located in the three lowest occupational categories (Dex and Walters, 1989). In France, too, 43 per cent of women are concentrated in five main occupations: secretarial, office work, sales, unskilled manual factory work and domestic cleaning (Mital, 1985). Even in Sweden, where a very high proportion of women work, segmentation of the labour market persists despite financial inducements to employers to take positive action to improve the situation – suggesting that cultural expectations of 'women's work' are remarkably resilient (Ruggie in Jensen *et al.*, 1988). Yet in spite of shared experiences of discrimination and inequality for women in Europe, there are particular characteristics of women's employment opportunities which, as suggested above, tend to place Britain in a poor light compared with most of its European partners.

Whether, and how, one should make judgements between states is very much the core of theoretical and practical debate in comparative studies. Whilst some commentators have argued against the use of general models to make such comparisons, others have sought to develop models or frameworks which encompass key indicators or features of societies and with which explanatory or analytical comparisons between different states can be made. (More recent examples include Bennett, 1990, Esping-Andersen, 1990; Mishra, 1990.) However, such models have disregarded gender issues in general (Dominelli, 1989; Langan and Ostner, 1991), and the working mother's perspective in particular, when assessing policy developments and/or outcomes. Drawing upon the most extensive study of child care and equality of opportunity for the EC (Moss, 1988), we are able to suggest features which might be added to existing models of social policy development and which may help to explain, or even classify, a particular country's stance in respect of women's welfare:

- the extent of publicly funded child care service
- employment adaptions to help employers reconcile family and work commitments.

Each of these key indicators could then be broken down into a series of more discrete criteria. The first, for example, might include both supply and demand subsidies, the amount and quality of state child care provision, the categories of children catered for, and the extent to which provision is flexible and offers choices for working and non-working mothers. The second indicator might well include the status ascribed to part-time work (as regards the right to part-time work as well as the rights of part-time workers), provision for parental and paternity leave, leave for family reasons, compensation for lost earnings, guarantee of job reinstatement, and, once again, the extent to which employers are able to offer choices to parents in employment. A further, third indicator of a country's position on women's welfare could be the state's role in providing equal opportunities for education, training and career progression.

If indicators such as these were incorporated into the models of welfare development currently available, the categories of welfare states thus identified may well have to be restructured, and the analysis and judgements flowing from such classifications re-examined. As Langan and Ostner (1991) point out, for example, Esping-Andersen's analysis of the 'de-commodification of labour' under different welfare systems quite excludes a gender dimension. It appears therefore that 'individuals who are commodified or de-commodified are all essentially similar'. Moreover, his use of Sweden as an exemplar of a social democratic welfare state, and his selection of evidence to demonstrate that it is also a decommodified state, have to be reconciled with the continuing gender bias in the labour market in Sweden, including within the public service sector (Wise, 1991) and between the public and private sectors (Langan and Ostner, 1991). Similarly, models of welfare which focus upon decentralisation as a point of 'convergence' between states (Bennett, 1990) and as a positive and welcome development for welfare programmes in Sweden (Einhorn and Logune, 1986) also ignore the possibility that this will disadvantage women if they continue to carry the disproportionate burden of acting as the key resource.

By contrast, the USA, a 'liberal individualist' state, has in some respects been more successful in removing gender barriers in occupation and has seen a higher proportion of women reach senior management posts in both the public and the private sectors. This has been achieved partly by the creation of more jobs – not all of which are junk jobs – and partly by the implementation of the Affirmative Action Program (Johnson, 1990).

Meanwhile, at a more practical level, the identification of specific criteria for assessing working women's welfare allows us to make discrete comparisons between Britain and elsewhere.

ASSESSING THE WELFARE OF WORKING WOMEN

First there is the continuing problem that part-time work is exploitative work. Whilst there is nothing intrinsic to the nature of part-time work which requires lower rates of pay, limited career prospects, poor working conditions, etc., these nevertheless remain the natural accompaniments to part-time work in Britain. In 1945, 45 per cent of employed women in Britain were working part time and of the new jobs taken by women in 1986–7 three-quarters were part time (Sharp and Broomhill, 1988). Of other countries in the European Community only the Netherlands has had a higher proportion of all women's jobs as part time – 52 per cent, compared with 17 per cent for Italy (Buckley and Anderson, 1988), 22 per cent for France and 30 per cent for Germany (Dale and Glover, June 1989). Furthermore, by being the only EC country not to have endorsed the Social Charter, which proposes important changes to protect, in particular, part-time workers, the government in Britain has done little to signal to employers the need to improve the status, pay and conditions of part-time women workers (*Guardian* 15 January 1991; *Poverty*, Winter 1990/91).

Second, caring responsibilities combined with lack of child care and other day care facilities, plus the consequent need for many women to stop working altogether, continue to present a major problem in Britain. As regards the care of young children, the UK lacks any clear coherent policy in respect of working parents. The current attitude is that child care generally is a private matter for the family (Moss 1989). Indeed, in terms of international comparisons, the UK is getting further behind other industrialised countries on this issue (Cohen, 1990a). But this approach militates against a comprehensive policy and could put the UK at a disadvantage in the European market after 1992.

Not only is the extent of childcare provision limited in Britain (e.g. in 1985 there were places for only 25 per cent of 0–4 year olds in public and private nurseries; (Brown, 1989), but much of the available day care is not actually designed to cater for the needs of working mothers. Likewise nursery education is designed not to meet the needs of mothers for child care but rather to serve the educational needs of the child – and most of it is part time. Even full-time provision is limited to the short school day and to school terms. Unlike the case with *écoles maternelles* in France, there is no provision for an extended day. Playgroups provide even more limited cover, generally offering only two or three half-day sessions a week and sometimes requiring the mother or father to attend.

The UK is, in fact, unique to the extent that it is the only country in the European Community where the majority of children in public nurseries are not there because their mothers work (Moss, 1988). Scarce nursery places are targeted on 'at risk' children from potentially abusive or neglectful homes or those who face other difficulties. In other words, so far as centre-based care is concerned, the UK appears unable or unwilling, by contrast with other European countries, to combine provision for the intellectual/social needs of children and the 'care needs' of parents. Although children start school at 5 years, the short school day and long holidays mean that even the part-time working mother is likely to need after-school care; but there is very little available (Cohen, 1990b) despite a recent government initiative designed to encourage it.

Comparative evidence on day care for children is particularly instructive, revealing as it does the UK as a relatively poor provider. Elsewhere, raising female labour force participation is invariably linked to plans for the expansion of day care, although provision is organised and financed in a number of different ways. The USA, for example, relies primarily on private market provision whereas in France and Scandinavia the public sector predominates. State subsidies can also be targeted on places and/or families in different combinations. Even so, in general, the highest levels of female labour force participation are linked to the extensive provision of state-subsidised nurseries (Brown, 1989). In Denmark, for example, where 80 per cent of mothers with children under 10 years work, 46 per cent of 0–2 year olds and 61 per cent of 3–6 year olds are in public day care. The private sector can also contribute, but the costs for parents of obtaining quality day care are high. To counter these costs, tax relief within the EC is available in France, Netherlands and Luxembourg (Moss, 1988).

Tax relief (demand subsidy) and public provision of places (supply subsidy) are not necessarily alternatives. France is an example of a composite approach. There is a traditionally high level of day care provision (95 per cent of 3–5 year olds were in *écoles maternelles* in 1988, many with an extended day provision, and 25 per cent of 0–2 year olds were in nurseries; Brown, 1989). But in addition France also provides tax relief on child care, and generous parental leave, so that families are presented with real choices.

Benefits which are everywhere closely tied to women's position in the labour market are maternity/paternity benefits and associated provisions for leave. The UK offers a comparatively long period of maternity leave of 29 weeks, longer than most OECD countries (Rutherford, 1989), but provides earnings-related benefit for a comparatively short period of 6 weeks (Wintour, 1990b). It is also of limited availability, requiring two years' continuous work with the same employer, of at least 16 hours a week, which means it will seldom be available after the second or subsequent births. By contrast, mothers in the US have no statutory right to maternity leave or pay but many employers make their own provision and about two-fifths of American women are in fact covered. Furthermore, the US does provide personal tax relief for day care, so in terms of a total package it is hard to determine relative superiority (Dex and Shaw in Hunt, 1988).

In the context of the EC and parental leave, Britain most certainly compares unfavourably with other countries by making no provision, thus highlighting its failure to relate labour market policies to family policy. Indeed, it has vetoed an EC Directive on parental leave on the grounds that this is a matter for individual employers. However, as many commentators make clear, it is impossible to separate inequality at work from inequality at home; so that, if equal opportunities are to be truly advanced through flexible work arrangements, parental leave would have to be high on the policy agenda. The Swedish system of parental insurance, an initial 12-month leave entitlement to be shared between both parents and an annual child sick leave entitlement, is generally regarded as a model of its kind (Hurstfield, 1987). But nearly every other country in the EC apart from Britain makes *some* provision for parental leave.

There is also the increasing need to pay attention to a broader dimension of caring that incorporates older, as well as younger, dependants. Whilst the average length of women's career breaks for child care has been reduced in recent years, the potential burden of caring for parents and grandparents looms larger as more people live longer and as official community care policies emphasise the centrality of informal care. In a study in Newcastle upon Tyne, 10 per cent of actual or potential returners to work were caring for older dependants (Hardill and Green, 1989). Yet a recent study found no private firms offering any support for elderly care (New Ways to Work, 1990b). Barclays Bank has since announced a policy of emergency care leave for its employees, allowing them up to five days of unpaid or 'borrowed' leave a year to care for elderly or ill relatives (*Guardian* 4 January 1991). In the USA, by contrast, a number of employers have introduced leave to care for elderly and ill relatives, while others offer computerised referral and assistance schemes for the community care of elderly patients (Wolcott, 1990). One company, Stride Rite, has even introduced the first inter-generational day care centre for the care of both children and elderly parents (Meade-King, 1990).

Finally, it is important to note the continuing underlying discrimination against women workers, irrespective of their family and caring responsibilities (Walby, 1988). On the basis of unproven assumptions that women lack commitment and ambition, employers in Britain have excluded them from access to inservice training (Homans, 1989), and discriminated against them for promotion purposes by using a range of career criteria which are not appropriate for many women, e.g. having an unbroken full-time work pattern, and being willing to be mobile and work outside normal hours (Harding, 1989). Those who take maternity leave are seen as automatically less dedicated to their employment, are denied training opportunities (Harding, 1989), and stand little chance of being assigned to the 'golden pathway' leading to rapid promotion (Homans, 1989). There remain, too, types of occupations and areas of work where both unions and employers are slow to relinquish their male preserve. This is well illustrated in the case of British Rail, an equal opportunity employer, which employs 20,000 train drivers of whom a mere 10 are women (Nevill *et al.*, 1990). These traditional attitudes towards women are deeply ingrained in many places of work and may not be easy to winkle out, even when a credible equal opportunity policy is in place. Evidence of the persistence of gender segregation in employment (see above p. 113) even suggests that there may be a measure of implicit collusion here between the expectations of employers and those of women themselves, mutually conforming to traditional stereotypes.

Opening training opportunities to both sexes is not enough in the face of a long history of discrimination. Educators and trainers blame one another, in a futile cycle, for the lack of any substantive change in women's job choices. The French have appreciated the need to be more active. Under the *Loi Roudy*, the Ministry for Women attacked blockages in schooling and training and ran a series of campaigns such as 'Let's Go Women' and 'Eliminate the Obstacles' designed to change social attitudes (Jensen *et al.*, 1988). For equal opportunities, it is argued, part-time training is as important as part-time work (EOC, 1981). Educational policy in Sweden has also taken a more positive line in breaking down gender stereotypes than has that in the UK, with the latter's largely token gestures of woodwork for girls and cooking for boys. It has to be admitted, however, that, even with commitment, progress can be slow in this area.

Too often, paid work and care work are seen as alternatives for women, and too infrequently do men share responsibilities for caring. Equal opportunities for women depend on broad family policies that seek to modify the role of men. As Brannen and Moss have concluded, measures taken by employers which are 'concerned with parenthood should be seen as needed by and applicable to both men and women' (Brannen and Moss, 1988: 162). This point has been grasped in Sweden, which has adopted a combined strategy incorporating benefits in cash and kind and flexible employment for parents of both sexes (Swedish Working Party Report, 1986). Esler also argues, with reference to Germany, that greater financial protection and higher status for reproductive work might induce men to take a greater share of it (Esler in Jensen *et al.*, 1988). The emphasis on flexibility for both men and women is the key to redeeming most part-time or flexible work in Britain from being a low-status, low-paid female ghetto.

It is in the context of these continuing major obstacles to effective equal opportunities and choices for women that we now turn to examining more specific and recent attempts to encourage women back to work.

RETURNER AND RETAINER POLICIES IN PRACTICE

A number of points may be made at the outset about such policies in Britain. First, even though they are driven by macroeconomic and employer needs, rather than by concerns for social justice, nevertheless they do represent an important development in furthering equal opportunities for women. They are a potential turning point in the long road towards real choices for women and men who have family commitments and who need, or want to work: 'Returner schemes constitute one of the ideal vehicles for the effective management of changes that are required by employers to meet the skills shortages of the 1990s' (Rajan and van Eupen, 1989).

Second, where policies are unfolding into good practice, these will be examined with interest by other employers both in Britain and elsewhere who are anxious not to be left behind in the search for more skilled personnel. As regards working women in other countries, where the opportunities for part-time work are traditionally more limited than in Britain, there is evidence that some women would actually prefer more flexible arrangements as long as these remain protected in respect of pay and conditions (Mital, 1985). If, for example, taking a break is a positive benefit for women, we should seek not only to preserve the option but to extend it to other workers, including men. There is firm evidence from both home and abroad that most mothers prefer to combine work and parenting (Moss and Fonda, 1980). For instance, a research study in Newcastle of middle-class and working-class mothers revealed a desire by both groups to spend some time raising their children. Brown also argues that there are positive reasons why some mothers do not work (Brown, 1989). In Denmark most mothers remain in the labour market after childbirth (Moss, 1989) but research has shown that 80 per cent of Danish mothers would prefer to work part time (Brown,

1989). Thus, despite cultural differences concerning paid employment for mothers with young children, there is no apparent rejection of the role of parent. So, if the examples of flexible work patterns now being offered to mothers in Britain prove successful, there may be some welcome opportunities for 'lesson learning' both ways. Job sharing, for example, which appears to be a peculiarly British development, is already attracting international interest (New Ways to Work, 1990b).

On the other hand, it is important to note, as the Institute of Manpower Studies study has indicated, that these flexible job opportunities are all relatively new ventures and still limited to a minority of employers, a mere 14 per cent in 1989 (Rajan and Van Eupen, 1989). Another survey undertaken in 1989 showed that, of all respondents, only 3 per cent of employers had introduced a childcare scheme, 8 per cent had established career breaks, and 7 per cent a job share scheme (Parson, 1990). Indeed, there is continuing evidence of considerable reluctance on the part of employers to adjust their recruitment policies and work structures in order to attract staff (*Guardian,* 10 April 1989). It has been suggested that good schemes not only provide flexible job arrangements to allow for family responsibilities, but also offer training and development for career advance and a clear corporate commitment to implement these policies. The rhetoric is often impressive: 'You can work full time, part time or on a flexible contract . . . on an arrangement that is right for you' (WMA, 1990). But the IMS claim that the real challenge to accommodate the career aspirations of returners has yet to be faced, and that the emphasis is currently still on the 'corporate image as a good employer' (Rajan and Van Eupen, 1989), rather than on the potential returner.

At least for some time to come, the reality for most British women is to leave and re-enter employment. In doing so they have a number of needs concerning education, training and job placement (EOC, 1990; WMA, 1990). They not only face problems of skills obsolescence, but also lack self-confidence in dealing with the world of work. Returners need not only competence but 'comportment' (Chalude and Liessein-Norman, 1987). If they have been out of the labour market for some years, they will have developed and matured as people and may well be looking for new job opportunities requiring new skills. According to Chalude, guidance and motivation courses are the first and indispensable form of assistance for many such women. Brown (1989) argues that we need 'not only to open the door but to help women through' and believes that information and counselling should not be attached only to compulsory re-entry. Access to courses is often restricted however, to those registered as unemployed, as is also the case in Denmark. Moreover training allowances are restricted. Chalude sees the allowance as having a psychological importance in awarding official 'permission' to attend, but it also broadens access. The Working Mothers' Association, for example, runs back-to-work workshops for women returning after career breaks but, at a cost of £95 for the day, it does little to encourage a wider take-up (WMA, 1990). Then again, careers guidance and practical advice are available, but from a bewildering variety of sources, as the EOC pamphlet *Signposts* for would-be returners makes clear (EOC, 1990).

Chalude *et al.* argue that cultural models in each country about how these forms of advice and support are offered will legitimately be different; but they stress that financial subsidies, to either business, training bodies or women themselves, are a necessary spur to action in any context. A number of polytechnics and colleges are now offering returner courses and they too emphasise the change in nature of the clientele in recent years, from middle-aged women who have raised their families and are looking for employment largely out of interest, towards younger women driven more by the need to contribute to the family income. Both the needs and the expectations of these groups are likely to differ, and, because women will seek re-entry at different ages and with diverse expectations, they are likely to need a range of different teaching styles (Davies, 1990).

Access to training is also important in facilitating a return to work. A recent Newcastle study showed that access to training, together with provision of child care, were the strongest factors helping women returners and that two-thirds of the women interviewed would like to learn new skills or update old ones. The authors claim that the demand for further training and its potential in facilitating return were the clearest findings in the study (Hardill and Green, 1989). An increasing number of firms are now offering refresher courses as an aid to recruitment. Many Health Authorities, for example, are running 'Come Back to Nursing' courses (Homans, 1989). The Commercial Union will 'help you learn new skills and refresh those that may be a little rusty', while Leicester City Council runs both returner and re-entry schemes for a wide range of staff linked to extensive opportunities for retraining. Tesco is experimenting with a 10-week returners' programme combining classroom techniques and live work experience designed to rebuild confidence (WMA, 1990).

Concerning the problem of skills obsolescence (though some writers have contested this assumption for women returning to their original employers – e.g. Gwartney-Gibbs in Guleh *et al.*, 1988), the IMS report identifies three ways of reducing the problem: first, regular contact during breaks, offering, for example, short refresher courses or short job spells; second, structured career counselling; and, third, formal education and training. A number of UK firms have recently offered retention packages to female employees (Rajan and Van Eupen, 1989; WMA, 1990). These link 'career breaks', commonly up to five years, with opportunities to work for a number of weeks a year, attend refresher courses and keep in touch through organised networks. One example is Littlewoods, which allows a five-year break during which there are opportunities to keep up to date with changes in the job role, attend internal courses, and short-term employment during peak trading times. Boots, the Electricity Council and a number of national clearing banks have also devised similar schemes to prevent skills obsolescence. Another example is Marconi, which allows an employee in engineering to take up to five years off work, during which time she is paid a retainer intended to cover the costs of journals and membership of professional associations. However, a recent survey undertaken by the IMS revealed that less than 0.01 per cent of women included in their study had benefited from any such career break (Metcalfe, 1990).

Job sharing, whereby one full-time job is split between two people, rather than job splitting, when two part-time jobs are created, is advocated by some as offering better opportunities for career advancement and for breaking down gender segmentation of the labour force (EOC, 1981; New Ways to Work, 1990b). Job sharers, unlike part-timers, are covered by equal pay and employment protection legislation. Moreover, job sharing is making inroads into areas of work which have been traditionally full time, e.g. staff nurse posts in the NHS, and management posts in industry. In the private sector, two companies in Britain, Boots and British Telecom, have taken a lead in offering a job share scheme (New Ways to Work, 1990b) and other companies, recognising the importance of flexible work arrangements, are now beginning to follow their example. Yet so far these provisions apply to only relatively few workers. The IMS study, for instance, found that only 2 per cent of employees were involved in job sharing (Metcalfe, 1990). A survey undertaken by The Industrial Society, which covered 20 large organisations, found only 6 of them offering job share, 'including one in which it is offered but not encouraged' (Nevill *et al.*, 1990: 72). Job-sharing policies have been offered by many London borough councils (New Ways to Work, 1990b), but, as a recent unfair dismissal case made clear, even these are ineffective if not adequately implemented (New Ways to Work, 1990a).

Other variations on the part-time theme are term-time working schemes, favoured by retailers like Littlewoods and Tesco's (WMA, 1990), and introduced recently by the Alliance & Leicester Building Society (New Ways to Work, 1990a). This option appears to be peculiar to the UK, but perhaps this is because after-school care is even more rudimentary than pre-school provision – unlike the situation in Sweden, Italy, France, Belgium or West Germany (Moss, 1989).

Technological developments make more feasible one form of flexible working which is especially attractive to employers as it involves very few capital overheads. This is home working, or, to use the more recent term for the new developments, teleworking. This pattern of working is likely to account for about 15–20 per cent of the total workforce in the UK (Hardyment, 1990). It may also help working mothers to look after their own children. The freedom to adjust work schedules, however, can also mean isolation and, apart from a small group of professional women, it can represent a low-pay, poor conditions ghetto for women, and a poor substitute for adequate child care provision (Hardyment, 1990; Hadsley, 1990).

If flexible working hours are to be offered by employers as part of a package to attract women back to a conventional working day, then childcare provision is obviously a critical issue. Day care frees women to work but it is often necessary for day care to free women to train first; failure to make this initial link can prevent women even getting to first base (Chalude and Liessein-Norman, 1987). The Newcastle study referred to above (Hardhill and Green, 1989) found that 78 per cent of the women interviewed considered child care an essential precondition for involvement in training. Given economic constraints, it is argued, the lack of day care will not prevent women from working but will confine them to a low level of flexible jobs constantly 'fitting round' children (Elias and Purcell in Hunt, 1988). The gap between demand for day care and the limited public supply is partially filled by child minding, but there is substantial evidence that, for many mothers, this represents a least favoured possibility, albeit often the only one available. Continental experience also suggests that most mothers favour group-based care (Kamerman and Kahn, 1981). In itself child minding also represents one of the most exploited sectors of female employment.

The other main alternative is commercial nurseries. Private nurseries in Britain have grown so rapidly recently (50 per cent over the last three years) that the Government has recently announced its intention of introducing new national guidelines drawn up by the National Children's Bureau (Berliner, 1990). Employers, also in a bid to secure women's labour, have turned their attention to nursery provision. Some have set up their own creches or undertaken joint ventures with other employers, or yet again purchased places in commercial nurseries for their employees. In the 1990 budget, Britain's government removed the tax burden from employer-based child care, but there is still evidence that employers are reluctant to get involved in direct provision, despite recognition that the current childcare situation is not conducive to women employees' recruitment or retention. The IMS study of retainer/returner schemes in Britain indicates that employers who are already offering flexible packages in terms of hours and conditions of employment tend to be only *thinking* about introducing creches (Rajan and van Eupen 1989). Direct childcare provision is their least preferred option (Industrial Relations Services, 1990).

Child Care Vouchers Ltd have put together a personalised voucher system which, it is argued, offers benefits to the employer in terms of aiding recruitment and emphasising commitment to staff welfare, yet with a minimum of administrative burden and a promise of tax benefits. To the mother they offer choice and childcare advice facilities (WMA, 1990). The organisation currently has 10 major clients (Meade-King, 1990). A government inter-departmental working group has recently endorsed the idea and it is suggested that it might soon be included in the budget (Wintour, 1990a). Such an approach might also be combined with provision of an information service along the lines of Child Care Link in Brighton – a child- care information and development centre which provides computerised information on day care vacancies in all sectors, and offers advice to parents. It is supported by the local authorities and sponsored by a number of large employers (Kulkarni and Sillence, 1990). This initiative, prompted by a labour shortage, is based on the American model of Resource and Referral Centers.

Those women who at the moment are most sought after by employers and who are therefore offered supported career breaks, childcare facilities, job share and flexible hours are those with scarce skills (Casey and McCrae, 1990). There is also evidence that those with higher initial levels of training are least likely to become de-skilled (Elias and Purcell, in Hunt, 1988). A key strategy, therefore, for effective retention and return must be to improve the basic education and training of the majority of women. While Armstrong argues that women's educational achievements now compare favourably with those of men (Armstrong and Armstrong, in Jensen *et al.*, 1988), it is still true to say that women continue to make restricted career choices and are under-represented on a wide range of training courses for skilled trades. The fact, as previously indicated, that this is so even in countries as committed to equal opportunities as Sweden, reinforces the contention that attitudes and expectations are so deep-rooted that change will require concerted policies bridging home, school and workplace.

CONCLUSION

It is difficult not to dwell on the obstacles to improving opportunities for women who want to work, and to concentrate on how little progress has yet been made in offering more flexible working arrangements which will better suit their needs. However, since we began by introducing a potentially optimistic perspective on current events in Britain, it is appropriate that we at least try to end on a more positive note.

First, from an employer's point of view there is much to gain. A recent British survey suggests that many UK employers have yet to realise the benefits of attracting women returners in the context of labour market shortages (Hardill and Green 1989). US cost–benefit calculations might favour less complacency. Intermedics Inc., for example, found that childcare centres reduced labour turnover by 23 per cent and helped absenteeism to drop (Wolcott, 1990). And in Britain, too, there is some small evidence that employers are beginning to recognise the benefits for themselves in offering career breaks (*Financial Times*, 22 February 1989). Thus, the more employers recognise the benefits of adopting flexible arrangements the more likely these are to secure a foothold.

Second, as we noted above, there has been some criticism of the role of the EC in the past. But a number of commentators are optimistic about the pressure the EC brings to bear on individual member states. Buckley and Anderson (1988) have noted, for example, that, whilst it remains primarily an economic Community, it has nevertheless made an important contribution to research, policy and practice concerning state commitments to equality of opportunity. Hoskyns (1985) has also noted that 'European initiatives are beginning to impose a common level of legislative provision on these issues throughout the Community' and, most important, she argues that 'it makes more difficult . . . attempts to weaken the position of women in the labour market'. One important recent example is the EC Directive on mandatory rules for minimum protection, which includes minimum pay. In the context of meeting its Social Charter commitments, the European Commission has proposed a new action programme on equal opportunities for women and men for 1991–95, which gives further scope for optimism. What is especially important is that the proposal singles out the need to develop new schemes to assist women with vocational training, qualifications and employment opportunities. It also makes special mention of the importance of developing childcare facilities.

Third, men as well as women are beginning to recognise the advantages for themselves of more flexible work patterns and sharing care responsibilities. That they can be as economically productive, if not more so, by adjusting their work habits now becomes more of a possibility thanks to technological developments. 'Flexilives', to use Handy's term, is clearly an idea whose time has come. 'Now, for the first time of our human experience, we have a chance to shape our work to suit the way we live instead of our lives to fit our work' (Handy, 1990: 141). As the Equal Opportunities Commission makes clear (1988: 5), one of its overarching objectives is 'To develop awareness and acceptance . . . that equal opportunities affects all aspects of men's and women's working and non-working lives'. It 'brings advantages to us all'. If, then, as we have suggested above, men are persuaded of the benefits of changing work patterns, continued pressure for further flexibility between working, family and personal life could be that much more attractive.

Yet there is the need for caution in interpreting such developments and the need, therefore, for vigilance. Even Professor Handy's optimistic perspective on working lives retains the expectation that it is women who will want 'bits of paid work' to fit into their portfolio, and to be 'paid' for their currently unpaid caring work. There is not too much emphasis here on men taking up unpaid caring work. Moreover, as Pahl (1988) notes, this is decidedly an alternative positive vision for managers and the 'middle-class salaried', not for those whose experience of home working amounts to exploitation and who have very few options in any domain.

Existing policies concerning reintegration of women in the labour force are riddled with contradictions. Currently they appear economically desirable, so employers support them but on their own terms and only while they feel the pressure of an acute skilled labour shortage. The government remains equivocal and so support for working women remains minimal. This is largely because, as Millar (1989) argues, the UK still starts from the assumption that mothers are normally at home, whereas other countries, especially in Scandinavia, assume that they will be working. Until perhaps the majority of women and men in Britain publicly register a preference for working (and caring) over not working, the ambivalence towards working women will ensure there is no policy direction towards an integrated approach involving training, day care, flexible conditions of employment and financial incentives. Whether intended or not, the consequence will be that qualified and experienced women will continue not to find employment consistent with their abilities (Main in Hunt, 1988).

Jensen *et al.* (1988) argue that women's situation is neither an eternal fact of nature nor a permanent social construct, but will depend on political action. The state, according to Sharp and Broomhill (1988), is not just a tool of capital, but can and has supported women. Thus there is scope for translating recent gains into lasting achievements. The evidence elsewhere of successful intervention by the state to support flexible options for women and men, both within the home and in the workplace, suggests that policy objectives shaped more by social justice than by the interests of the economy are both legitimate and feasible. Considerable political effort will be required to safeguard recent improvements, but this can be made in the knowledge that more choice in both work and domestic life is an achievable goal.

REFERENCES

Beechay, V. and Perkins, T. (1987) *A Matter of Hours. Women Part-Time Work and the Labour Market*, Cambridge: Polity Press.

Bennett, R. J. (1990) *Decentralization, Local Governments and Markets*, Oxford: Clarendon Press.

Berliner, W. (1990) 'Starting out strongly', *Guardian*, 24 April.

Brannen, J. and Moss, P. (1988) *New Mothers at Work*, London: Unwin Hyman.

Brown, J. (1989) 'Why don't they go to work? Mothers on benefit', *SSAC Research Paper 2*, London: HMSO.

Buckley, M. and Anderson, M. (eds) (1988) *Women, Equality and Europe*, Basingstoke: Macmillan.

Casey, B. and McCrae, S. (1990) 'A more polarised labour market', *Policy Studies* VII (2), Summer.

Chalude, M. and Lissein-Norman, N. (1987) *The Re-insertion of Women in Working Life*. Luxembourg: Commission of the European Communities.

Cohen, B. (1990a) *Caring for Children. The 1990 Report*, London: Family Policy Studies Centre.

—— (1990b) *Guardian*, 7 November.

Dale, A. and Glover, J. (1989) 'Women at work in Europe', *Employment Gazette*, June.

Davies, C. (1990) 'Working towards change', *Health Services Journal*, 25 October.

Dex, S. and Walters, P. (1989) 'Women's occupational status in Britain, France and the USA: Explaining the difference', *Industrial Relations Journal* 20 (3), August.

Dominelli, L. (1991) *Women across Continents*, London: Harvester-Wheatsheaf.

Einhorn, E.S. and Logune, J. (1986) *Modern welfare states. Politics and Policies in Social Democratic Scandinavia*, New York: Praeger Publications.

Employment Gazette (1989) 'Labour force outlook in the year 2000', April.

—— (1990) 'Women in the labour market', December.

EOC (1981) *Job Sharing – improving the quality and availability of part-time work*, Manchester: Equal Opportunities Commission.

—— (1988) *From Practice to Policy*, Manchester: Equal Opportunities Commission.

—— (1990) *Signposts*, Manchester: Equal Opportunities Commission.

Esping-Andersen, G. (1990) *The Three Worlds of Welfare Capitalism*, Cambridge: Polity Press.

Guleh, B., Stomberg, A. and Harwood, S. (1988) *Women and Work. An Annual Review*, Vol. 3, Sage.

Hadsley, N. (1990) *Guardian*, 19 December.

Halsall, M. (1990) 'A workforce raring to go if someone would let it', *Guardian*, 24 September.

Handy, C. (1990) *The Age of Unreason*, London: Arrow.

Hardill, I. and Green, A. (1989) *An Examination of Women Returners in Newcastle*, University of Newcastle on Tyne.

Harding, N. (1989) 'Equal opportunities for women in the NHS: the prospects of success? *Public Administration* 67, Spring, 57–63.

Hardyment, C. (1990) 'Staying at home for the quietest revolution of all', *Guardian*, 27 January.

Health Services Management (1989) Editorial, August.

Homans, H. (1989) *Women in the National Health Service – report of a case study on equal opportunities in clinical chemistry laboratories*, London: HMSO.

Hoskyns, E. (1985) 'Women's equality and the European Community', *Feminist Review*, 20 Summer.

Hunt, A. (1988) *Women and Paid Work*, London: Macmillan.

Hurstfield, J. (1987) 'Part timers under pressure', London: Low Pay Unit.

Huws, V., Hurstfield J. and Holtmaat, R. (1989) 'What price flexibility? The casualization of women's employment', London: Low Pay Unit.
Industrial Relations Services (1990) 'Effective ways of recruiting and retraining women', August.
Jensen, I., Hagan, E. and Reidy, C. (1988) *Feminization of the Labour Force*, Cambridge: Polity Press.
Johnson, R.A. (1990) 'Affirmative action policy in the United States: its impact on women, ' *Policy and Politics* 18 (2).
Kamerman, S. (1983) *Maternity Policies and Working Women*, New York: Columbia University Press.
Kamerman, S. and Kahn, A. (1981) *Child Care, Family Benefits and Working Parents – A Study in Comparative Policy*, New York: Columbia University Press.
Klein, R. and O'Higgins, M. (eds) (1985) *The Future of Welfare*, Oxford: Blackwell.
Kulkarni, J. and Sillence, G. (1990) 'Making Child Care Links. Report on the setting up of the Brighton Project'.
Labour Research (1990) 'Narrowing the pay group – UK women lag behind', March.
Lane, C. (1989) 'From "welfare capitalism" to "market capitalism" a comparative review of trends towards employment flexibility in the labour market of three major European societies', *Sociology* 23(4), November.
Langan, M. and Ostner, I. (1991) 'Gender and welfare' in G. Room (ed.) *Towards a European welfare state?*, Bristol: SAUS/SPA.
McCrae, S. (ed.) (1990) *Keeping Women in*, London: Policy Studies Institute.
McLaughlin, E. (1989) 'Work and welfare benefits', paper presented to Social Policy Association Conference, summer.
Meade-King, M. (1990) 'Who cares about working mothers', *Guardian*, 3 July.
Metcalfe, H. (1990) *Retraining Women Employees – measures to counteract labour shortages*, Institute of Manpower Studies, Report No. 190, April, University of Sussex.
Millar, J. (1989) *Poverty and the Lone Family: Challenges to Social Policy*, Avebury.
Mishra, R. (1990) *The welfare state in Capitalist Society*, London: Harvester Wheatsheaf.
Mital, C. (1985) 'Quand les femmes travaillent', *L'Expansion*, October/November.
Moss, P. (1988) *Child Care and Equality of Opportunity*, London: European Commission.
—— (1989) 'Child care and employment', paper presented to Social Policy Association Conference, summer.
Moss, P. and Fonda, N. (1980) *Work and the Family*, Uxbridge: Brunel University, Maurice Temple Smith.
Nevill, G., Pennicott, A., William, J., and Worrall, A. (1990) *Women in the Workforce*, London: The Industrial Society.
New Ways to Work (1990a) *New Ways to Work Newsletter* 6(3), London.
—— (1990b) *Pioneering New Work Patterns – Annual Report*, London: New Ways to Work.
Pahl, R. (ed.) (1988) *On Work*, Oxford: Blackwell.
Parson, D. (1990) 'Winning workers', *Employment Gazette*, February.
Rajan, A. and Van Eupen, P. (1989) *Good Practices in the Employment of Women Returners*, Institute of Manpower Studies Report, University of Sussex.

Rutherford, F. (1989) 'The proposal for a European directive on parental leave', *Policy and Politics*, 4, 301–10.

Sharp, R. and Broomhill, R. (1988) *Short Changed, Women and Economic Policies*, London: Allen and Unwin.

Swedish Working Party Report (1986) *The Changing Role of the Male*, Stockholm.

Walby, S. (ed.) (1988) *Gender Segregation at Work*, Milton Keynes: Open University Press.

Weston, C. (1990) 'Firms improve terms to keep women staff', *Guardian*, 4 October.

Wintour, P. (1990a) 'Minister supports creche voucher plan', *Guardian*, 9 July.

—— (1990b) 'Britain lags on maternity leave', *Guardian*, 19 July.

Wise, L. Recascino (1991) 'Internal labour markets in civil service systems. A framework for comparative analysis', Conference on Comparative Civil Service Systems, 17–19 October, Leiden/Rotterdam, The Netherlands.

Wolcott, T. (1990) 'The structure of work and the work of families', *Family Matters*, April.

WMA (1990) *Returners' Guide – a practical guide for women returning to work*, London: Working Mothers' Association.

Part III
Prospects for Europe

7 Towards a European welfare state?

On integrating poverty regimes into the European Community

Stephan Leibfried

Who overcomes
By force, hath overcome but half his foe.
    (John Milton, *Paradise Lost*)

EUROPEAN INTEGRATION AND SOCIAL POLICY: HISTORICAL AND ANALYTICAL APPROACHES

Europe is more than just a geographical entity. And it is more than a 'common market'. Europe has a common tradition in war, peace, culture and, above all, welfare statism – making it a distinct peninsula on the Asian continent (Schulze, 1990). The legally still separate West European nations may be about to merge into a United States of Europe ('USE') or at least into a steadily increasing 'pool' of 'shared sovereignties' – an economic, political as well as cultural entity of its own – analogous to but also quite different from the USA. This process and prospect has been gaining momentum during the past two decades. After several unsuccessful attempts, the Single European Act of 28 February, 1986 and the Maastricht summit of December 1991 have moved the European Community (EC) closer to an economic, a political, and to some extent also a social union.[1] By now, the EC has definitely developed beyond just a 'tariff union' – but where is it moving? Will there be a European welfare state, a 'transnational synthesis' (Offe 1990: 8) of national welfare states, with 'European social citizenship' being one backbone of the USE? Or will the welfare state, which is 'characteristic only for this part of the world' (van Langendonck, 1991), be irrelevant for 'building the new European state'? Will fragmented 'social citizenships' remain at the national level, where they might slowly erode? (c.f. Majone, 1992)

If European unification were not to be based on 'social citizenship', European welfare regimes would remain at the USE's state or 'regional' level and stay below the supranational level of visibility. The regimes of poverty policy, the most exposed parts of social citizenship, would then be most likely to corrode slowly and inconspicuously. This may cause phantom pain for social welfare and, in particular, poverty experts. In their respective national contexts they would be struggling with the consequences of something that never came to be: a European welfare state built on a European poverty policy.

The options and constraints involved in building a European welfare state constitute the topic of this paper. I will focus mostly on European poverty regimes and will discuss them historically and typologically.

From negative to positive integration

If 'European social citizenship' or 'Social Europe' is to come about, a 'positive' mode of integration is required. Such an integration is much more ambitious and complex than a pure and simple 'common market' goal. It aims at joint 'constructive' action, at a 'positive state'. However, the evolution of 'prefederal' European institutions, of Europe's 'incomplete federalism', has been strongly moulded by 'negative integration'. (A summary of the two modes of integration is given in Table 7.1.) Negative integration focuses on 'deconstruction', on just removing obstacles to a free market, thus being unmindful of inherent social consequences (Kaufmann, 1986: 69).

Moving from 'freedom' to 'social rights' implies a shift in the nature of the political regime in a unifying Europe[2] – a shift from negative to positive integration. The discussion on 'Social Europe', on the 'social dimension', on the 'Social Charter', and on some details of the EC social policy mandate is already testing the limits of the unification regime of the European Community. In this context, the poverty issue is of special relevance, since it is morally clear cut and marks the 'North–South' divide in the Community itself. To address European poverty the EC would have to design programmes which aim at all European families. However, the EC mandate is focused mostly on European employees and their families – and not yet on the European citizen *per se*. Even the EC Social Charter refers mostly to employees,[3] although comparable basic statements of rights at the national level address all citizens.

Interestingly enough, the negative integration modus of the EC was transcended (mostly) in agricultural policy in the Rome Treaty at the very start of European integration (Pinder, 1968:100f.). In the European Community, as well as in the USA, agriculture was the first 'internal' policy domain to be 'nationalised'. This has fundamentally affected the development of a supra-national bureaucracy in the USA (Skowronek, 1982; Dupree, 1957; Rossiter, 1979) and at the EC level this development also incorporated different social policy developments, at first only vis-à-vis

Table 7.1 Types of integration

Modus of integration	*Nature of tasks*	*Political system*	*Examples in present EC legislation*	*Classical and typical models*
Negative	Rremove obstacles	Weaker; strong reliance on juridical procedures and decisions	Free movement of persons, goods, capital, and services (*the four freedoms*)	'Tariff Union' ('Zoll Verein') (Germany before 1871 or USA; Italy?)
Positive	Create common social space	Stronger; reliance on a developed executive and parliament	Set minimum of essential health and safety requirements	'German *Reich*' (after 1871), Canada.

Note: See Dehousse (1988:313) on the first three columns.

agriculture. More attention should be paid to how universal social welfare components might be systematically intertwined with the agricultural domain at the EC level, and not only to how a 'basic income' for certain agricultural producers is or might be achieved EC-wide. The US Food Stamps programme might offer a modest example of such a process. Since the EC has been granted legal and administrative competence in this area, it might at first be easier to widen these established policy channels,[4] rather than struggling for a comprehensive EC social policy based on positive integration.

Historical models for European integration in the social policy domain

Two major examples highlight the different relevance of 'positive integration' or 'social unification' for processes of national integration:[5] the German unification of 1871 – and again of 1990 – and the consolidation of a United States of America as a 'state' at the turn of the twentieth century.

The German Reich

The first German integration of 1871 did not conform to the 'normal' (Anglo-Saxon) pattern of evolution of rights, i.e. one expanding from civil to political to social rights (cf. Marshall, 1964). The extension of social citizenship to the working class – not to the poor *per se* – which was the core of Bismarck's social legislation, preceded political citizenship (that is, introduction of universal suffrage after defeat in World War I) by four decades.

Integration of the German Reich – as in England – was mainly achieved through social reform. 'One nation' grew out of a class-divided 'two nations' in a sphere of common social rights. An overdose of social citizenship, mostly granted to men, as well as a homogeneous national bureaucracy,[6] was administered to a nation about to unify – hence identifying the (mostly male) 'Second Nation', or the organised working class, with the new, benevolent national state, the 'social security state'. The new welfare state of the 1880s became the foremost intermediary (not directly state) bureaucracy,[7] which legitimated an otherwise fragile central government.

Today's German unification repeats, compressed in time, the pattern of 1871: civil and social unification preceded the political union, though – contrary to 1871 – the chances of an improved 'integration through social reform' have been mostly bypassed by (West) German politicians.[8]

At first, the German Democratic Republic (GDR) seemed to aim at a synthesis of the 'social advantages' of West and East Germany and proposed a 'Social Charter'. But in the meantime, the West German social policy model has simply been extended (sometimes in a watered-down version) to the territory of the former GDR, in some cases allowing for transition periods, and now making it 'the' German model. There may be some lasting consequences of German social unification in the area of minimum income legislation, since transitional minimum pensions and minimum unemployment benefits have been provided for in the Unification Treaty. Many issues which had pointed towards the need for a new era of social reform during the unification period, and which had been 'displaced', resurface now that unification is implemented. West German policy solutions often do not fit reality in the five new states. So 'social cohesion' is an important inner-German issue, which is triggering compensatory action but not comprehensive social reform.

In any case, German unification today will be viewed by others – especially in Europe's southern countries, its Latin rim, and in Ireland – as a leading case for 'integration' policy.[9] Perhaps unification can contribute to changing Germany's role in the EC in a positive way, too, with Germany now more inclined to promote European social unification instead of blocking it as it did in the past. Other EC countries, especially at the Latin rim, will closely monitor the German 'integration experiment'; it may become a 'regional observatory' for a possible development of the social dimension of the EC.

USA

In the USA, the historical sequencing of 'citizenship' is 'normal'. This Anglo-Saxon pattern conforms to the one we can also observe in the EC: first come civil, then political, and then social rights. The USA thus offers the best counter-example to the German Reich of 1871: it operates with an 'underdose' of social rights – instead political and civil rights are strongly emphasised. Vis-à-vis the EC, the USA offers a good comparative case, since it shares central features: both 'continents' are unified through 'federations', and the unification of both is court-led and court-fed, [10] with juridification playing a central role. At the turn of the century, the USA was still just 'a state of courts and parties' (Skowronek, 1982) – thus a non-state at least in the European sense. On the other hand, the EC might be characterised as a 'state of the European Court and of Brussels technocrats'.

Social policy in the USA was at first only indirectly nationalised. Long before the Great Depression of the 1930s, two classical Departments – War[11] and Agriculture[12] – incorporated social policy functions. Until the Great Depression the national level was otherwise void of social policy competencies, a situation which was first altered by Roosevelt's introduction of social security. The historical legacy of this gaping hole in national social responsibility is a permanently labile state of nationalisation of social policy itself, which today is seen best in 'functionally decentralised' US poverty policies.

Viewed from the perspective of a USE-to-be, the EC is now confronted by a similar 'void'. Will the nations of Western Europe be able to cope with this challenge of 'social cohesion' faster and more successfully in the twenty-first century than the USA was able to in the twentieth century?

The EC versus the USA and the German Reich

The USA – like the EC, but in contrast to the German Reich – has stayed closest to the 'tariff union' pattern, the typical model of negative integration. At the same time, the USA has a more highly integrated political structure than the EC might ever achieve. In Table 7.2, differences in federal developments of the USA and the EC are contrasted. For the USE and the USA, there are different fault lines. In the USA the fault line runs between political and social rights, since a 'common market' and a political union have developed there in one process. In the sequence of citizenships, social citizenship comes last. The USE, though, has two such fault lines: the same one as in the USA, but also a preceding one that runs between civil and political rights. A European synthesis will thus be especially demanding. The situation of the EC therefore resembles the development in the USA less

Table 7.2 Types of federalism and lines of breakage: the USE versus the USA

	USE	USA
Type	Incomplete federalism	Complete federation
Market ('*civil citizenship*')	Common market	Interstate commerce
Parliamentary Governance etc. ('*political citizenship*')	Political union	Congress, federal government
Welfare state ('*social citizenship*')	Social union, '*Social Europe*'	Broad federal powers for social regulation
Remarks	Rome Treaty left competency vacuum in social policy and provided for meagre forms of political representation; no EC social citizenship (needle's eye: employment relationship: atrophy of national social citizenship regimes, e.g. welfare, child allowances, youth welfare, housing allowances, etc.)	With the Great Depression, the competency vacuum at the federal level was filled by redefinition of constitutional powers.

Note: Fault lines= === and ▬▬

than it looks like the building of the German Reich of 1871 – at that time, Germany also had to deal with two such fault lines at once. But Germany dealt with social citizenship earlier than it did with political citizenship. This reversal of the sequence is also of interest for an analysis of European integration marked by a distinctly lagging 'political union'.

When we look at the EC compared with the USA or the German Reich this question arises: should and will EC development conform more to the Anglo-Saxon pattern of sequencing citizenship or to the German one? In the former case, European unification would take place without a social foundation but would rest, on the contrary, on a market-oriented foundation of 'possessive individualism'. In the latter case, European unification would instead attempt a synthesis of civil, political and social rights thus confronting both fault lines at once and breaking with the Anglo-Saxon pattern of development. 'Social Europe', 'social dimensions' of European development, a 'Social Charter' (Kommission, 1989; Silvia, 1991; Addison and Siebert, 1991; Bercusson, 1989; Lange, 1992), 'Social Fund'[13] – at the moment these are catch-phrases in symbolic politics pointing at a social foundation without really building any of the structural prerequisites. Only a confluence of several favourable conditions will contribute to a breakthrough for a truly Social Europe.

THE FOUR SOCIAL POLICY REGIMES IN THE EC

We have seen that positive integration, 'social cohesion', is not built into the present structure of the EC. There is no EC welfare state (outside of agriculture). If we look at the different existing welfare systems in Europe may we then realistically expect that a 'Social Europe' will come about by an 'organic' merging of such systems from the bottom up? Positive integration at the EC level would then be a by-product of ongoing European economic and political integration. Or are the social and poverty policy regimes of the EC so contradictory that an organic merging from below is not possible and 'harmonisation' will necessarily have to come 'from above', i.e. it will have to be synthesised and implemented by an authorised EC bureaucracy? Such a European welfare state would, most likely, presuppose a historical North-South compromise within the EC and, surely, a reformulation of the Rome Treaties, partly already achieved in Maastricht. Without an EC welfare state, in the long run, regional, national welfare regimes will be in atrophy: their economic and legitimatory bases would slowly erode with the completion and further development of the Common Market – just as they eroded in the USA with the realisatian of its 'common market' interstate commerce (Peterson and Rom, 1990).

Whether Social Europe might come about via merging from the 'bottom up' can be examined by reviewing typical EC poverty regimes. My attention will centre on the interfaces between poverty, social insurance and poverty policy. The different consequences which the introduction of a *basic income* scheme under each regime might have will be outlined.[14] This is one way to illustrate the practical importance of the differences between these regimes.

Though the discussion of welfare state regimes usually focuses on those policy areas that quantitatively dominate the welfare state – i.e. the social insurance systems (cf. Schmidt, 1988) – I concentrate on the margins of the welfare state; it is here that the limits – and the contents – of social citizenship are tested, and it is here that any differences in European social policy will be most obstructive.

In the following, I will distinguish four different social policy regimes – four 'worlds of welfare capitalism':[15] the Scandinavian welfare states, the 'Bismarck' countries, the Anglo-Saxon countries, and the 'Latin rim' countries.

The Scandinavian welfare states

Since World War I, the welfare states of Scandinavia[16] have stressed the right to work for everyone and have centred their welfare state policy on this issue and not on compulsory income transfer strategies. Scandinavia fits the type 'modern welfare state'. Universalism reigns, though not primarily through income redistribution outside the sphere of work. Here, the welfare state is *employer of first resort* (mainly for women). Subsidising 'entry' into – or non-exit from – the labour market is the welfare state strategy which conveys the institutionalised notion of social citizenship.

In Scandinavian countries, the basic income debate is likely to be used only as an additional argument for the support of a universalist 'work-centred society'. The debate might be of some use for improving 'income packaging' in the Scandinavian welfare state (see Rainwater *et al.*, 1986). Broad-scale issue-specific redistribution, like child allowances, might be improved. Or the rather residual, truly marginal welfare systems there might be improved in such a way that they match the standards of 'Bismarck' countries. But basic income is unlikely to develop into a strong option; to opt out of 'work society' as a general strategy will not be condoned.

The 'Bismarck' countries

For a century, Germany and Austria have relied on a strategy of 'paying off' social problems, of subsidising 'exit' from the labour market or even 'non-entry' while pursuing a strong policy of economic development only. These countries might be characterised as 'institutional welfare states'. Here, 'compensatory strategies' which substitute a right to social security for a right to work are prominent, and a basic income debate would be most likely to radicalise the present focus on compensation and exit (or non-entry). The welfare state is not the employer but the *compensator of first resort*, and the institutionalised notion of social citizenship is biased accordingly. Though there is no explicit tradition of universalism in these countries, the 'institutionalised full employment promises' and private labour market 'practices' (of the 1950s to the early 1970s) have created a fragile tradition of virtual universalism (for an overview cf. Leibfried and Voges, 1992).

The basic income debate here amplifies the pre-existing focus on non-entry or easing-exit from the labour market. Perhaps in the Bismarck countries this debate could lead to something like a universalised non-residual needs approach which might become less and less restrictive in terms of means-testing and might also develop towards an individual instead of a household orientation.

The Anglo-Saxon countries

The English-speaking countries have always emphasised the 'residual welfare model' (see Titmuss, 1987: 262), especially in income transfers.[17] They did not accent, as the Scandinavian countries did, the welfare state as the major employer in a 'work society'; rather, they conceived of the welfare state as a work-enforcing mechanism (see Lødemel, 1989). The USA, Australia, New Zealand, and also the UK best exemplify the type of 'residual welfare state' (Titmuss, 1987: 367). 'Entry' into the labour market was facilitated more by pure force than by subsidisation or by training and qualification policy. Here, selectivism reigns as the principal approach of social policy, making the welfare state rather a *compensator of last resort*. The distance of the Anglo-Saxon model from a 'compensatory regime' or from a Scandinavian 'work society regime' is equally great. Thus 'social citizenship' has remained more of an academic issue in these countries.[18]

The basic income debate in the Anglo-Saxon countries is rather far away from institutionalising an 'option out of work society'; it may support the development of a 'normal welfare system' in the Northern European sense. However, the development is not likely to go any further than this. A normal welfare system in the Anglo-Saxon context would mean (especially in the case of the USA) introducing a universal instead of a 'categorical' welfare system (treating each category differently), combining this welfare system with a more prominent role for a public jobs programme that aims at integration into the primary labour market (somewhere between the German and the Scandinavian model), and having adequate ('fair share') and nationally standardised (again especially in the case of the USA) 'welfare' rates.

The 'Latin Rim' countries

The southern countries of Western Europe, some of them integrated into the EC only in the 1980s, seem to constitute a welfare state regime of their own. This league comprises Spain, Portugal, Greece, to some extent (southern) Italy and, least of all, France.[19] This type could be characterised as 'rudimentary welfare state'. In Portugal, Spain, Italy and Greece, not even a right to welfare is given. In some respects, these states are similar to the Anglo-Saxon countries, *de facto* stressing residualism and forced 'entry' into the labour market. But in these countries, older traditions of welfare (connected to the Catholic Church) seem to exist on which the Anglo-Saxon model and most northern countries cannot build. Moreover, in these countries certain social security programmes serve as basic income measures, although they were not designed as such (the disability pensions in southern Italy seem to have worked out this way; see Ascoli, 1986: 113f., 122). In addition, labour market structures are radically different and often reveal a strong agricultural bias, combined with a 'subsistence' economy which provides a different – non-Northern European – 'welfare' state background. Finally, these countries do not have a full employment tradition – in particular, one that also fully applies to women – as do some of the Scandinavian countries. But many of these countries have made strong promises pointing towards a 'modern welfare state' in their constitutions; it is the legal, institutional and social implementation which seems to be lacking in the 'Latin Rim', the welfare state of *institutionalised promise*. It is hard to gauge the effect of a basic income debate in these countries. The development of 'normal welfare systems' seems most likely – normal in the sense of the Northern European or German welfare model.

These four types of welfare state are summarised in Table 7.3. Modern, institutional, residual and rudimentary welfare states start from rather different, in some cases contradictory, goals and are built on quite disparate intervention structures; and they do not share a common policy (and politics)

Table 7.3 Types of European welfare states

	Scandinavian	Bismarck	Anglo-Saxon	Latin rim
Type of welfare regime	Modern	Institutional	Residual	Rudimentary
Characteristics	Full employment; welfare state as *employer of first resort* and compensator of last resort	Full growth; welfare state as *compensator of first resort* and employer of last resort	Full growth; welfare state as *compensator of last resort* and tight enforcer of work in the market place	Catching up; welfare state as a semi-*institutionalised promise*
Right to:	Work	Social security	Income transfers	Work and welfare proclaimed
	Backed up by an institutio-nalised concept of social citizenship		No such back-up	Implemented only partially
Basic income debate	Marginal, but may improve income packaging	May somewhat radicalise decoupling of work and income	May support development of 'normal' welfare system	May support development of normal welfare system

tradition that could serve as a centripetal force. In any case, this divergence of regimes does not lend support to the notion that a European welfare state might grow via automatic harmonisation, building from the national towards the EC level. A 'bottom up' strategy for EC 'social integration' policy seems stillborn.

WHITHER EUROPEAN WELFARE POLICY: 'Europeanisation' from the 'top down' or 'Americanisation' from the 'bottom up'?

What may be the influence of a continuous Europeanisation of economic and representational policy on social, especially poverty, policy? Since automatic harmonisation of European social policy, building from the national towards the EC level, is not likely, two alternatives remain:

1 Policy disharmony in welfare policy may either prevail as a permanent underside of European integration or, worse, be transformed into a process of automatic disharmonisation at the bottom. National politics may be 'Balkanised' as the European Common Market solidifies, especially when a common currency is achieved. This process resembles what happened to American poverty policy as the New American national state was built, starting at the turn of the twentieth century.

2 Policy disharmony may also provoke – in particular when confronted with more potent pressures for European 'social cohesion' – a Caesarian reaction of European institutions. This might prompt a comprehensive European policy frame for poverty policy – or for all social benefits – primarily tied to social citizenship. In the context of currency union some such non-incremental development is likely, if it is not prevented through advance incremental social state building at the EC level in the short time remaining in the 1990s.

Towards 'Americanisation' of European poverty policy?

In this part, I will concentrate on 'Americanisation' as one alternative. Since this path is closest to the given EC situation, I will show how it corresponds with present EC welfare legislation, which is mainly procedural and not substantive (see Table 7.4 below). The development of EC legislation again fits in with the historic model of evolution of poverty policy in European nation-states (see Table 7.5 below).

In my view, European development will most likely leave all poverty and welfare policy at the local or state – that is at a sub-European – level. It is hard to start from a common European denominator. The easy common ground is missing on which a European welfare regime could be built.

Table 7.4 Status, EC residence permit and poverty support in Germany

	Residence permit	Right to welfare
Self-Employed	For Economic activity within EEC treaty framework (freedom of services and capital movement); otherwise, see 'Others'	Yes; only take-up of welfare parallel to economic activity is legitimate; otherwise, take-up results in loss of right to residence and in possible deportation
Employed *Pre-employed:*	For job search in due time (according to EC law, 3 months)	Yes; beyond due time, take-up of welfare results in loss of right to residence and possibly in deportation[a]
Employed:	Even in the case of sub-poverty-level of remuneration	Yes; parallel take-up of welfare is legitimate
Unemployed:	cf. pre-employed; for the involuntarily unemployed, permit expires as 'availability for work' is denied[b]	Yes; when permit expires, take-up of welfare results in loss of right to residence and possibly in deportation
Not employed[c] *Students:*	If registered for study and insured in event of sickness	Only temporarily; costs may be recovered from 'home state' of recipient[d]
Pensioners:	If insured in event of sickness and in receipt of sufficient (old age, accident, disability) pension to avoid take-up of welfare	Yes; but take-up of welfare results in loss of right to residence and possibly in deportation
Others:	If insured in event of sickness and in receipt of sufficient resources to avoid take-up of welfare	Yes; but take-up of welfare results in loss of right to residence and possibly in deportation

Notes:
a   Section 10, para. 1, no. 10, Ausländergesetz (Alien Bill) stipulates that foreigners may be deported if they cannot support themselves without the take-up of welfare.
b   Section 103, AFG (Employment Bill).
c   In the following, I refer to legislation proposed by the Commission (see *Amtsblatt der Europäischen Gemeinschaften*, 28 July, 1989, Nr. C 191/2–6; KOM(89) 275 endg.-SYN 199, 200; 89/C 191/02–04). The Council of Ministers agreed to these somewhat modified proposals on 22 December, 1989 (cf. FAZ 23 Dec. 1989). As yet, the 'Not employed' have no mobility rights which are Community protected.
d   Such recovery, though, would contradict section 4 of the European Convention on Social and Medical Assistance, ratified by all 12 EC member countries.

In contrast to poverty policy, some work-centred social policies – 'health' and 'work safety' issues – would be much easier to 'Europeanise' or to 'harmonise', since these policies are structured in a fairly comparable way to begin with and since the European institutions have a stronger mandate there. Needs-centred social policies are rather difficult to standardise and will have no strong thematic lobby in the European context – unless some poor 'Latin rim' states make it a 'state issue' – and such policies will have a hard time finding a mandate. Thus, the most likely outcome is that needs-centred social policies are least likely to be protected by European development.

One might therefore predict that the 'Europe to be', in terms of social policy and especially in terms of poverty policy, will look much more like the USA did before the 1930s, or like it does today, than like any of the Northern European welfare regimes. Europe after 1992, as far as poverty policy is concerned, might lead to a shift towards the Anglo-Saxon welfare model; at least, it is likely to lead to a welfare state 'Balkanisation' quite similar to that in the USA. If 'integration' in poverty policy comes about within these limits it will be of a negative sort, allowing each member state to have its own regime and creating only procedural rules, perhaps also about how to proceed with 'foreign' recipients and with the re-exportation of their burden to their 'home' countries.[20]

What is the current state of EC welfare policy? The few EC rules on welfare that do exist are meaningful only in 'national welfare contexts', where they are meant to become operational. Therefore, I will discuss them in a national – in this case, the 'welfare state generous' German – setting.

At present the situation, as it is captured in Table 7.4, is still at a level where receiving welfare leads to the classic 'poor law' remedial procedures: ship the poor back to their place of origin (in the EC). The EC, therefore, compares with the evolution of poverty policy in European nation-states – still bound to the first of four historical and logical levels of integration of poverty policy, as shown in Table 7.5.

A second, more refined stage of social policy development is realised when a person is permitted to stay in the country granting him or her welfare but the costs of support are charged back to his or her place of origin (Table 7.5). To channel transfers from many national sources through one national agency is a regular feature of social security networks established in bilateral agreements; for example, when pensions are paid to an aged migrant worker. Community law allows for this possibility in welfare policy exclusively for 'students', a most temporary status (see Table 7.4: Not employed, *'students'*). An internal administrative shifting of costs is still rare between national poverty bureaucracies. At the moment, such a solution seems not to be envisioned for the aged (see Table 7.4: Not employed, *'pensioners'*) – though they are closest to pensioners, where this solution already exists within social

Table 7.5   Steps in integration of poverty policy

Step	Characteristics
1	'Shipping the poor back home'
2	Shifting only the costs of poor support to the locality of origin
3	Treatment of EC citizens as national (or local) citizens in each country (or community)
4	Creation of European substantive and procedural welfare standards

insurance. An aged person moving from Germany to Spain, therefore, has to prove to the Spanish authorities that he/she has sufficient resources not to be in need of welfare. Nevertheless, a solution similar to that for 'students' may have to come about for pensioners who did move to another EC country, stayed there for a long time, and then needed long-term care arrangements that they could not afford without welfare co-payments. Rather than destroy the new, last social roots at the place of retirement by insisting that these pensioners return to their country of origin in the EC, it would seem more desirable to recover outlays from that country.

A third step in the evolutionary ladder (see Table 7.5) is taken when take-up of welfare in Germany – or for that matter in any other EC country which grants a right to welfare – becomes as legitimate for EC citizens as it is for German citizens, or for the citizens of any respective EC country. This is the case only in connection with employment (see Zuleeg, 1987); most extremely in the case of low-wage employment (see Table 7.4: Employed, '*employed*'), less in the case of joblessness ('*unemployed*') and least in the case of non-employment (job search, '*pre-employed*').

The European Court decided in the cases of Levin and Kempf that it is only relevant under European law that a person be gainfully 'employed' and 'active in wage or salaried employment', independent of whether he/she is earning less than the state-defined subsistence minimum (Zuleeg, 1987: 344f.). For the residence permit of an EC citizen 'it is irrelevant whether such income . . . is increased by other income up to this minimum or whether the person is satisfied with his [or her] below-poverty income, as long as he [or she] is truly active in wage or salaried employment' (European Court Reports 1986, 1749ff.). This interpretation does not hinge on what the country concerned defines as 'employment'; it thus holds universally in the EC.

Thus German social security law – Section 8 of the fourth book of the SGB, the Welfare Law Code – levies no pension contributions on 'insignificant employment', defined as being below 15 hours per week or earnings less than 470 DM (parameters as of 1 January 1990).[21] Looking at the hours only, Kempf – the plaintiff in the European Court case – would not have been considered 'employed' according to German law. But according to superior EC law he is considered 'employed' in Germany, and thus has a right of residence and access to all social benefits in Germany, which includes a right to welfare.

Independent of what a national 'standard employment relationship' is, the EC and its courts set their own Europe-wide principles. A broad interpretation of 'employment' through the Court has been one of the avenues of moving towards 'social citizenship' under the constraints of an employment-oriented concept of freedom and European integration (see, most extensively, Steinmeyer, 1990). The same solution obtains in the case of self-employment that does not provide sufficient resources for self-support (see Table 7.4: Self-employed). Again, welfare may be legitimately used as a supplementary benefit for EC citizens. In this case, however, there is no 'pre' and 'post' protective status as it relates to the employment situation (job search, unemployment). Self-employment is thus less shielded in an EC social policy context against the risk of poverty. But there is also less of a necessity to shield it: empirically, these cases are not very significant; and legally, a Gestaltswitch of the 'self-employed' into the status of 'employed, searching for work' can easily be orchestrated by the person concerned.

The four steps in integration of European poverty policy have been summarised in Table 7.5. At present, Step 1 is still the norm, and Steps 2 and 3 are the exception. Step 4, which aims more at a European poverty regime, is entirely out of reach. If the European Court of Justice were to take up the challenge of the Maastricht revisions of the EC Treaty, this might catapult the EC's social and poverty policy immediately to Step 3 (Table 7.5) and would do away with all present residential and financial restrictions discussed above. Why? Because until now European citizenship has been limited to the migrant worker and – *through* him or her – to the family. But at the Maastricht summit, to demonstrate at least some headway in political and social union, it was agreed 'to strengthen the protection of the rights and interests of the nationals of its Members States through the introduction of a citizenship of the Union'. The agreement reads:

> Citizenship of the Union is hereby established. Every person holding the nationality of a member state shall be a citizen of the Union. Every Union citizen shall have the right to move and reside freely within the territory of the Member States [and to receive consular support. No explicit fiscal preconditions seem to be set.] Union citizens resident in the Member States of which they are not nationals will have the right to vote and stand as candidates in municipal and European elections.
>
> (*Financial Times*, 12 December 1991: 6)

This agreement may just seem symbolically gratifying. But it could actually imply for Europe what two basic Supreme Court decisions, Edwards v.

California and Shapiro v. Thomson, [22] achieved for the USA: a right to travel, even when the aim is just to attain better special social benefits.[23] Edwards was arrested for bringing his brother-in-law, an indigent, from Texas to California. To grasp the European analogy let me quote some of the Supreme Court's reasoning in 1941. While California pleaded that other states, like Texas, should not be able 'to get rid of their poor . . . by low relief and insignificant welfare allowances and drive them into California to become our public charges' (168), the Supreme Court focused on the limits which a federal union places on state power:

> And none is more certain than the prohibition against attempts on the part of any single state to isolate itself from difficulties common to all of them by restraining the transportation of persons and property across its borders. . . . [T]he peoples of the several States must sink or swim together, and . . . in the long run prosperity and salvation are in union and not in division. (174)

Central to that Supreme Court decision was an underlying assumption, an 'assumed *national* responsibility to address the problem of poverty' (Garth, 1986:100). The Supreme Court notes a 'growing recognition that in an industrial society the task of providing assistance to the needy has ceased to be local in character. The duty to share the burden, if not wholly to assume it, has been recognised not only by State governments, but by the Federal government as well' (175). From a federal point of view it does not matter whether poverty is in Texas or in California. Does it matter from an EC point of view whether poverty is in Portugal or in Germany, in Ireland or in England? The EC with its new competency vis-à-vis 'social exclusion' (*Financial Times*, 12 December 1991), with its new unconditional citizenship and its old general responsibility to deal with 'regional inequality' (Structural Funds), could grasp this opportunity for member states to swim instead of to sink together, if 'social citizenship' were to become a focus for a continuous rights-building exercise at the EC level from the 1990s onwards.

'Europeanisation' of poverty policy

European institutions could also define European standards of poverty policy, 'social rights' for European citizens 'from the top down' – in a Bismarckian, Napoleonic fashion. These standards could be designed to bring the top – the more generous welfare systems – down or to bring the bottom – the more miserly welfare systems – up. These standards could rely on a European formula (for example, 40 per cent of the average national wage income to be used as the basic welfare rate of each nation) which could still allow for variance between the different nations. As yet I do not see how the political and juridical base for a beneficial European standardisation might be forthcoming. However, if the EC may not set standards that inform a European right to welfare, it might still subsidise national poverty policy systematically; for example, in underdeveloped or peripheral regions (cf. on the different strategies, Hauser, 1983, 1987).

With social security 'harmonised' – or not (see Schmähl, 1989: 47) – at the national level and not institutionalised at the European level, it would be a rather peculiar situation to have poverty policy partly centralised supranationally at the EC level. The 'showcase' effect vis-à-vis the poor produced at the Community level might even surpass the national 'parading of the poor' so well known from the US social policy scene in AFDC (Aid for Families with Dependent Children).

The Europeanisation of poverty policy might also take quite a different angle: it may be that certain risks (the 'deserving poor') will be Europeanised; for example, the 'poverty of the aged' and, much less likely, the poverty of the unemployed.[24] Here, there might be an agreement among all nations for a rather positive means-tested solution. Thus, the 'deserving' categories of the poor, which are already 'privileged' in many of the EC member countries (see Schulte, 1991), could be Europeanised. All the other poor might be left to be dealt with at the state or local level according to diverging national traditions. This filtering of the poor might permit a cultural construction of an 'underclass' at the national level, a stratum against which prejudice might then be better directed.

If such a development were to come about, it would lead to another Anglo-Saxonisation (in the sense of the US model) of the European welfare context: the 'categorical' approach to welfare will be imported and the universal approaches which are dominant in Northern European states will be slowly subverted. The USA, with its fixation on single mothers' welfare (AFDC), is the most prominent example of the categorical approach – which Germany had already discarded in the 1920s. Also, if the EC decides partly to subsidise minimum income developments, then control devices of special revenue sharing, as they have evolved in the US residual welfare policy regime (especially in AFDC), are likely candidates for Europeanisation. Once the benefits of means-tested income transfers cannot be targeted at nationals only, such transfers may either slowly wither away or have to be delivered directly at the European level or nationally in a strongly harmonised way.

Since European Community law at present (some changes are under way) makes national solutions of the categorical sort difficult unless these nations allow 'transfer exports' to other European countries – the economic benefits of such transfers may not be sheltered nationally (Zuleeg, 1989) – there is a political and economic incentive for a straightforward European categorical solution.

That a more radicalised version of a basic income might become the European Community approach seems, at this time, rather unlikely[25] – though the discussion of these issues in a European context may be beneficial for a push towards more generous traditional 'welfare' solutions at the European level.

CONCLUSION

A unified European poverty regime is no 'all-purpose weapon'. Surely, Europe should develop its own perspectives on a 'War on Poverty' and its standards for a fair distribution of income. Poverty, though, is not limited to the income dimension alone but concerns all sorts of resources – be it education, qualifications, or other means of social integration (see Friedrich *et al.*, 1979:11–47). But to focus first on absent income may be the easiest way to make deprivation and marginalisation visible ('social reporting'; see Leibfried and Voges, 1990) at the European level and to politicise them, using it as an eye-opener for wider poverty issues.

Access to the road from a common market to a Social Europe, a European welfare state, has barely been gained. It will be a long road – but with monetary union on the books it may have to be travelled speedily (Eichengreen, 1990). Germany's first unification at the end of the last century led to the creation of the national welfare state. This state was built on a then timely concept of social citizenship – for workers. The founding of a United Europe depended mainly, if not totally, on the 'four freedoms': the free movement of persons, goods, capital and services. Thus 'economic citizenship', which does contain some civil aspects of 'social citizenship', [26] is at the fore. Political as well as social citizenship have, until now, been marginal in the process of European unification. For this reason, European unification reminds one more of the unification of the USA – a process in which political citizenship was pertinent from the beginning and has been complemented by social citizenship only since the 1930s, if at all.

The citizenship on which a unifying Europe might come to rest seems primarily an economic or civil notion, secondarily a political one, and only lastly a social one (see Marshall, 1964:78ff.). This pattern repeats British and American precedents and is not anchored well either in Germany or in Scandinavian history. Unity in such a restrictive frame would turn into a unity of 'possesive individualism', a unity of markets only. It will not be the unity of an enlightened 'Social Europe' synthesising its traditions of democracy and solidarity, of civil and social rights, and building on its traditions of merging the citizen and the social state. But, maybe, steps taken towards European citizenship at Maastricht in 1991 will allow the metamorphosis of the 'market citizen' (1957–91) into the 'full-fledged' EC citizen – a new synthesis which includes a European welfare state trajectory, building on universal rights?

The coming of such an enlightened 'Social Europe' also depends on the challenges provided and the escapes offered by its 'environment'. Japan and the USA do not offer the EC a better model for social integration. 'Social Europe' might lose much of its impetus if Eastern Europe – at least being perceived as 'social' pressure in the days of 'systems competition'[27] – were to turn into 'less Central Europe than *Zwischeneuropa* ... a dependent intermediate zone of weak states, national prejudice, inequality, poverty, and *Schlamassel*' (Ash, 1990: 22).

ACKNOWLEDGEMENTS

This paper is reproduced in edited and revised form, by permission of Campus Verlag of Frankfurt a.M. and Westview Press of Boulder, Colorado, from the volume *Social Policy in a Changing Europe*, edited by Szusza Ferge and Jon Eivind Kolberg, published May 1992 in the series 'Public Policy and Social Welfare'.
I am grateful to Lutz Leisering, Chiara Saraceno, Bernd Schulte, Peter Townsend and several participants at the 1990 annual conference of the Social Policy Association in Bath for comments and critical remarks. Hannah Brückner, Marlene Ellerkamp, Peter Klein, Jutta Mester and Gitta Stender were helpful in completing this paper.

NOTES

1 The 'social' component was already an issue between France and Germany at the time of the Rome Treaty, though not as a 'Social Union'. Then, the issue was: should social policy expenditures be counted as labour costs in establishing 'free markets'? Decades later, in the 1960s, the 'Social Union' re-emerged in attempts by the Commission to move towards harmonisation in social policy, which failed. Finally, in the early 1970s, another attempt was made for a 'European Social Union', supported by the German government headed by Willy Brandt. Herbert Wehner, head of the parliamentary SPD, envisioned 'the United States of Europe constituted as a democratic welfare state' (Vereinigte Staaten von Europa in der Form eines demokratischen und sozialen Rechtstaates). Cf. for an overview Henningsen, 1992.

2 The two regime types are not exclusive. The shift from negative to positive integration implies a synthesis: positive integration includes *and* transforms negative integration by relating to concepts of 'justice' and 'welfare'. Positive integration confronts the 'social infrastructure' necessary to achieve 'negative integration', thus not simply displacing the costs of integration downwards.

3 'Social' policy at the EC level is structurally narrow – it is usually understood as 'employment' policy only, i.e. programmes for those employed or employable. When Jacques Delors speaks about a 'social floor' for Europe he means not a floor for citizens but one for the employed only. The 'labourer' and the 'citizen' (in the nineteenth century, the 'poor') are treated as distinct social categories.

4   A not too successful version of this was tested in the extremely cold winter of 1987 when the European ministers for agriculture decided to have agricultural surplus products distributed to the needy at no cost. This programme has been continued since then (see Henningsen, 1989: 74) and costs more per year than the entire ('other') four-year poverty programme of the EEC. This programme was later discontinued.

5   At the time these developments took place they looked much more like 'supranational' integration. Only in retrospect and in the light of their success do they look like processes of mere 'national' integration.

6   German unification after 1871 was, compared with the US, not particularly influenced by agricultural interests. 'Poverty' and 'agriculture' were issues within one Interior Department. After World War I, the Reich's Labour Ministry (*Reichsarbeitsministerium*) evolved as 'the' social policy unit out of the Department of the Interior. Agricultural policy in Germany, in contrast to the US, had no pioneering role in the nationalisation of social policy competence.

7   The social security bureaucracies are not direct parts of the national German government or of the state governments. They are independent national or state agencies, usually of a corporatist nature, with their governing bodies staffed by representatives of labour, employers and the different levels of government.

8   If (West) Germany had accepted the challenge, a synthesis might have looked quite interesting. The German Democratic Republic's road to a welfare state differed substantially from the West German one: it guaranteed a right to work (and thus did not institutionalise unemployment insurance), with the labour force participation rate of women being far higher than in the FRG. Redistributive policies focused less on the aged – as they do in West Germany – than on the young. Social policy operated mainly through the provision of public goods. With respect to monetary transfers, uniform minimum approaches dominated. Thus had the GDR moved from the Bismarck model, which it had inherited, towards the Beveridge model.

9   In Germany, two countries were unified which were much further apart than the extremes within the EC. The differences between the FRG and the GDR in poverty, for example, are rather similar to the North–South incline obtaining in the EC; but in addition the whole economic system was at variance, which is not the case in the North–South incline of the EC.

10   The Supreme Court in the USA and the European Court in Strasbourg are the respective core of these integration processes.

11   In the Department of War, a strongly expanding pension system was built up after the Civil War. This system partly stepped in for a then not existing federal welfare state (Skocpol and Ikenberry, 1983).

12   At first, this was just social policy for the farmworkers, but with Food Stamps in the second half of the twentieth century the scope of social policy has been extended to the urban population. Food Stamps is still the only programme available to any poor person in the US and it is nationally uniform. The programme is administered by the Department of Agriculture, even though it is quasi-money (coupons) and not food which is distributed today (cf. Leibfried, 1992b).

13   Compared with the Social Charter, however, the Social Fund is a real institution, though its scope is modest. The Social Fund of the EC demands as much in terms of fiscal resources as do Child Allowances in former West Germany alone.

14   On the structure of 'Basic Income Security' in former West Germany see Leibfried, (1990a).

15 I add another category ('Latin Rim' countries) to Esping-Andersen's (1990) three worlds of welfare capitalism. I have studied potential trajectories of *'top down'* development of a European welfare state elsewhere (Leibfried, 1992a; Leibfried and Pierson, 1992).

16 In fact, the Scandinavian model is essentially a Swedish model, which holds for Norway, Denmark and Finland only with important modifications.

17 If one took in-kind transfers into account, the prominent UK example of the NHS would highlight the taxonomy in a different way.

18 This is, historically speaking, more so in the USA than in the UK, though England has moved visibly towards the US in the last decade.

19 In France (see Haupt, 1989: 271ff.) the strong family focus of all social policy (and concomitantly of wage policy) probably leads to a special sort of welfare state regime.

20 Outside of building social insurance institutions against poverty in old age or with regard to invalids and the sick, this was the traditional pattern of poverty policy integration in the building of the German Reich from 1871 to World War I. The 'Unterstützungswohnsitzgesetz' basically left all substantive poverty law to the states or local governments and was concerned only with issues of 'free mobility'.

21 The same holds true for health insurance. Blue-collar workers working less than 10 hours a week have no right to continued wage payments in the event of sickness. Then again, unemployment insurance does not reach out to certain 'part-time employed'. For instance, it covers only people working 18 hours and more per week.

22 394 US (1969). The Supreme Court dealt here with statutes which limited welfare benefits to persons who had resided for at least one year in the respective state. Justice Brennan: 'State may no more try to fence out those indigents who seek higher welfare benefits than it may try to fence out indigents generally' (631).

23 'Social tourism' is the not so benign label in the negative political discourse that is characteristic of Northern Europe looking south (and lately east).

24 In the 1970s an EC initiative to partly 'Europeanise' unemployment insurance was blocked by the Council (Taylor, 1983: 223). The 'Study Group on Economic and Monetary Union' (Marjolin Report) had proposed a European component to national unemployment insurance in 1975. The MacDougall Report (1977) had given this proposal further momentum. The Council blocked this initiative in 1978. Both reports stressed the fact that a common currency would be an inescapable 'forcing mechanism' for the EC. Since national governments would lose most of their traditional adjustment instruments (devaluation, deficit spending), only the EC at the supranational level could then deal effectively with regional inequality and social cohesion – unemployment insurance and regional (infrastructure) policy being amongst the most suitable instruments here. A similar case might be made for unemployment insurance *and social assistance* in tandem. The EC currency union of the 1990s will most likely ensure proposals such as these resurface soon.

25 At the European level, basic income is unlikely to become a means to opt out of politics and socio-political issues since, for example, there is no European consensus whatever on building an institutional welfare state at this level which could legitimate simply 'paying off' social problems.

26 Only those aspects of Marshall's civil citizenship are captured that pass the needle's eye of 'free mobility'. Freedom of speech, thought and faith, for instance, would play a minor role; the right to own property and to conclude valid contracts, and the pertinent right to justice, would play a major role.

27 The necessity to 'outcompete' East Germany in social policy was behind much of West German social reform in the 1950s. On this 'struggle of principles' see Hockerts (1980). This necessity has now withered away. In its stead 'functional equivalents', internal mechanisms, will have to be developed which serve as forcing mechanisms for social innovation in the future.

REFERENCES

Addison, J.T. and Siebert, W.S.(1991) 'The Social Charter of the European Community: Evolution and Controversies', *Industrial and Labor Relations Review* 44 (4), 597–625.

Ascoli, U. (1986) 'The Italian Welfare State between Incrementalism and Rationalization' in Laura Balbo and Helga Nowotny (eds) *Time to Care in Tomorrow's Welfare Systems: The Nordic Experience and the Italian Case*, Vienna: Eurosocial, 107–141.

Ash, T.G. (1990) 'Eastern Europe: The Year of Truth', *New York Review of Books*, 15 February, xxxvii (2), 17–22.

Bercusson, B. (1989) *Fundamental Social and Economic Rights in the European Community*, Florence: EUI.

Dehousse, R. (1988) 'Completing the Internal Market: Institutional Constraints and Challenges'; in Roland Bieber, Renaud Dehousse, John Pinder and Joseph H.H. Weiler (eds) *1992. One European Market? A Critical Analysis of the Commission's Internal Market Strategy*, Baden-Baden: Nomos, 311–336.

Dupree, A.H. (1957) *Science in the Federal Government: A History of Policies and Activities to 1940*, Cambridge, Mass: The Belknapp Press of Harvard University Press (reprinted 1986).

Eichengreen, B. (1990) 'One Money for Europe? Lessons from the US Currency Union', *Economic Policy* 10, 117–187.

Esping-Andersen, G. (1990) *The Three Worlds of Welfare Capitalism*, Cambridge: Polity Press.

Friedrich, H. *et al.* (1979) *Soziale Deprivation und Familiendynamik*, Göttingen: Vandenhoeck and Ruprecht.

Garth, B.G. (1986) 'Migrant Workers and Rights of Mobility in the European Community and the United States: A Study of Law, Community and Citizenship in the Welfare State', in Mauro Cappelletti, Monica Secombe, Joseph Weiler (eds) *Europe and the American Federal Experience, Vol. I: Methods, Tools and Institutions, Book 3: Forces and Potentials for a European Identity*, Berlin: de Gruyter, 85–163.

Haupt, H.G. (1989) *Sozialgeschichte Frankreichs seit 1789*, Frankfurt a.M.: Suhrkamp.

Hauser, R. (1983) *Problems of Harmonization of Minimum Income Regulations Among EC Member Countries*, Frankfurt a.M., sfb 3, Working Paper no. 118.

—— (1987) *Möglichkeiten und Probleme der Sicherung eines Mindest-einkommens in den Mitgliedsländern der Europäischen Gemeinschaft*, Frankfurt a.M., sfb 3, Working Paper no. 246.

Henningsen, B. (1989) 'Europäisierung Europas durch eine europäische Sozial-politik?' in Peter Haungs (ed.) *Europäisierung Europas*, Baden-Baden: Nomos, 55–60.

—— (1992) 'Die schönste Nebensache Europas – Zur Geschichte der EG-Sozialpolitik', *Sozialer Fortschritt* 41(9), 204–12.

Hockerts, H.G. (1980) *Sozialpolitische Entscheidungen im Nachkriegsdeutschland. Alliierte und deutsche Sozialversicherungspolitik 1945 bis 1959,* Stuttgart: Klett-Cotta.

Kaufmann, F.X. (1986) 'Nationale Traditionen der Sozialpolitik und Europäische Integration' in Lothar Albertin (ed.) *Probleme und Perspektiven Europäischer Einigung,* Cologne: Verlag Wissenschaft und Politik, 69–82.

Kommission 1989: *Kommission der Europäischen Gemeinschaften, Generaldirektion Beschäftigung, soziale Angelegenheiten und Bildung, 1989: Soziales Europa, Der Kampf gegen die Armul* (Social Europe. The War against Poverty), Brussels, Luxembourg: Publications Division of the EEC, 100 pp. (CE-NC-89-002-DE-C).

Lange, Peter (1992) 'The Politics of the Social Dimension' in Alberta M. Sbragia (ed.) *Europolitics, Institutions and Policy Making in the 'New' European Community,* Washington DC: Brookings Institution, 225–56.

Langendonck, J. van (1991) 'The Role of the Social Security Systems in the Completion of the European Market', *Acta Hospitalia* no. 1, 35–57.

Leibfried, S. (1990a) 'Soziale Grundsicherung – Das Bedarfsprinzip in der Sozial und Gesellschaftspolitik der Bundesrepublik', in Georg Vobruba, (ed.) *Strukturwandel der Sozialpolitik. Lohnarbeitszentrierte Sozialpolitik und soziale Grundsicherung,* Frankfurta. M: Suhrkamp, 182–225.

—— (1990b) 'Sozialstaat Europa? Integrationsperspektiven Europäischer Armutsregimes', *Nachrichtendienst des Deutschen Vereins für öffentliche und private Fürsorge* 70 (9) September, 296–395.

—— (1992a) 'Social Europe, Welfare State Trajectories of the European Community', in Hans-Uwe Otto and Gabi Floesser (eds) *How to Organise Prevention,* Berlin: de Gruyter, CeS-Working Paper No. 10/91, 17–60.

—— (1992b) 'Nutritional Minima and the State – The Institutionalization of Professional Knowledge in National Social Policy in the US and Germany', Bremen: CeS – Working Paper No. 10/92.

Leibfried, S. and Pierson, P. (1991) 'The Prospects for Social Europe', *Politics & Society* 20(3), 333–66.

Leibfried, S. and Voges, W. (1990) 'Keine Sonne für die Armut. Vom Sozial-hilfebezug als Verlauf ('Karriere') – Ohne umfassende Information keine wirksame Armutsbekämpfung', Nachrichtendienst des Deutschen Vereins für öffentliche und private Fürsorge 70 (5), May, 135–41.

—— (eds) (1992) *Armut im modernen Wohlfahrtsstaat,* Opladen: Westdeutscher Verlag.

Lødemel, I. (1989) *The Quest for Institutional Welfare and the Problem of the Residuum. The Case of Income Maintenance and Personal Social Care Policies in Norway and Britain 1946 to 1966,* London: LSE, Department of Social Science and Administration, June.

MacDougall Report (1977) *Report of the Study Group on the Role of Public Finance in European Integration, Vol. 1: General Report, Vol. 2: Individual Contributions and Working Papers,* Brussels: Commission of the European Communities, Economic and Financial Series A 13.

Majone, G. (1992) 'The European Community between Social Policy and Social Regulation', Florence: European University Institute, unpublished manuscript.

Marjolin Report (1975) *Report of the Study Group 'Economic and Monetary Union 1980',* Brussels: EC, March.

Marshall, T.H. (1964) 'Citizenship and Social Class' in T.H. Marshall, *Class,*

Citizenship and Social Development, Essays by T.H. Marshall, with an introduction by Seymour Martin Lipset, Chicago IL: University of Chicago Press: 71–134.

Offe, C. (1990) 'Europäische Dimensionen der Sozialpolitik', Bremen: Centre for Social Policy Research, July, unpublished manuscript.

Peterson, P.E. and Rom, M.C. (1990) *Welfare Magnets*, Washington DC: Brookings Institution.

Pinder, J. (1968) 'Positive Integration and Negative Integration – Some Problems of Economic Union in the EEC', *World Today* 24, 88–110.

Rainwater, L., Rein, M. and Schwartz, J. (1986) *Income Packaging in the Welfare State: A Comparative Study of Family Income*, Oxford: Clarendon Press.

Rossiter, M.W. (1979) 'The Organisation of the Agricultural Sciences', in Alexandra Oleson and John Von (eds) *The Organisation of Knowledge in Modern America 1860–1920*, Baltimore, MD: Johns Hopkins University Press, 211–48.

Schmähl, W. (1989) 'Europäischer Binnenmarkt und soziale Sicherung – einige Aufgaben und Fragen aus ökonomischer Sicht', *Zeitschrift für die gesamte Versicherungswirtschaft*, 29–50.

Schmidt, M.G. (1988) *Sozialpolitik. Historische Entwicklung und internationaler Vergleich*, Opladen: Leske and Budrich.

Schulte, B. (1991) 'Das Recht auf Mindesteinkommen in der europäischen Gemeinschaft. Nationaler status quo und supranationale Initiativen', *Sozialer Fortschritt* 40(1) 7–21.

Schulze, H. (1990) *Die Wiederkehr Europas* ('The Reform of Europe'), Berlin: Siedler.

Silvia, S.J. (1991) 'The Social Charter of the European Community. A Defeat for European Labor', *Industrial and Labor Relations Review* 44 (4), 626–43.

Skocpol, T. and Ikenberry, J. (1983) 'The Political Information of the American Welfare State in Historical and Comparative Perspective' in Richard F. Thomasson (ed.) *The welfare state 1883–1983*, Greenwich, and London: JAI Press, (Comparative Social Research, vol. 6) 87–148.

Skowronek, S. (1982) *Building a New American State. The Expansion of National Administrative Capacities, 1977–1920*, Cambridge: Cambridge University Press.

Steinmeyer, H.D. (1990) 'Freizügigkeit und soziale Rechte in einem Europa der Bürger' in Siegfried Magiera (ed.) *Das Europa der Bürger in einer Gemeinschaft ohne Binnengrenzen*, Baden-Baden: Nomos, 63–80 (this approach is discussed on pp. 81–7).

Taylor, Paul (1983) *The Limits of European Integration*, New York: Columbia University Press.

Titmuss, R.M. (1987) 'Developing Social Policy in Conditions of Rapid Change: the Role of Social Welfare', in Brian Abel-Smith and Kay Titmuss (eds) *The Philosophy of Welfare. Selected Writings of Richard M. Titmuss*, London: Allen and Unwin, 254–68 (First published 1972).

Zuleeg, M. (1989) 'Die Zahlung von Ausgleichszulagen über die Binnengrenzen der Europäischen Gemeinschaft', in *Deutsche Rentenversicherung*, no. 10, 621–29.

Zuleeg, S. (1987) 'Zur Einwirkung des Europäischen Gemeinschaftsrechts auf die Sozialhilfe nach dem Bundessozialhilfegesetz', *Nachrichtendienst des Deutschen Vereins für öffentliche und private Fürsorge* 67 (10), 342–7.

Zuleeg-Feuerhahn, S. (1992) 'Berucksichtigung von Kindererziehung in der Rentenversicherung, das Territorialitatsprinzip und das Europäische Gemeinschaftsrecht', *Zeitschrift fur Sozialreform* 38(10), 568–88.

8 The end of the middle way?

The Swedish welfare state in crisis

Arthur Gould

INTRODUCTION

Until recently it looked as if the power of Swedish social democracy would escape the more extreme reaction which has been experienced by other welfare states. After six years of bourgeois party rule between 1976 and 1982, the Social Democratic Workers' Party (SAP), was returned to office and went on to win the general elections of 1985 and 1988 with its proportions of the popular vote hardly changed. While in the UK a Conservative government rejected Keynesianism, extensive state welfare, a strong public sector and the commitment to full employment, Sweden not only clung to them, but seemed to maintain a strong record of economic growth. Representatives of the Labour Party in the UK continued to visit Sweden well into the 1980s to find out how the Swedes did it. In 1991, however, it was beginning to look as though the middle way had come to a dead end. Economic growth was −0.5 per cent, living standards were declining, and unemployment was on the increase. Major cuts were being made to welfare services and benefits and support for the SAP in public opinion polls had sunk to a consistent all-time low. The conservatives were within a few percentage points of becoming the largest of Sweden's political parties and would be fighting the general election in September 1991 on a clear neo-liberal platform.[1]

THE WELFARE STATE

The foundations for the Swedish welfare state were established when the SAP took office in 1932. Major social programmes to alleviate unemployment and provide financial support to families led Marquis Childs to describe Sweden as 'The Middle Way', by which he meant that the country had successfully combined the better features of both capitalism and socialism (Childs, 1936). Two years after Child's book appeared, the

Swedish federation of manual workers' trade unions (LO), was reaching a basic agreement about pay levels for the coming year with the employers' association (SAF). This historic compromise coupled with another, support by the Agrarian Party (now known as the Centre Party) for the social democrats, provided a firm basis for economic growth and the expansion of social programmes for many years to come. Neutrality in World War II meant that the economy was not only protected from devastation but thrived on opportunities for exporting to those nations engaged in combat. Impressive growth rates continued into the 1940s and 1950s and the government began to establish major national programmes for health, pensions and housing. By the 1960s, Sweden was becoming the world leader in state welfare not only in the cost, range and quantity of its programmes but also in their quality and resourcefulness. Few visitors to the country came back with anything but praise for the way the impressive wealth of the economy was helping to create not only private affluence but public affluence as well. Tomasson described Sweden as the prototype for a modern society – a model for others to follow (Tomasson, 1970). It was organised, clean, efficient. Poverty did not seem to exist. It was difficult to find fault with the way in which the People's Home was being run.

By the 1970s Sweden had a universal system of health insurance, income-related old age pensions, sickness benefits amounting to 90 per cent of income, a comprehensive system of schooling based upon mixed-ability teaching, an active manpower policy and a formidable, high-quality housing programme. Looking back it was interesting to see how the Swedes had developed a consensual approach to their social policies. Looking forward, it was invigorating to see what they anticipated for the future.

Most of the major reforms had been accomplished by the government setting up a commission to investigate a particular social problem. These commissions would deliberate for a number of years – often 10 or more. During this time they would set up research programmes, establish experimental projects and come up with proposals which would be sent out on *remiss* to all interested parties. At the end of this long process the government would invariably seek the views of opposition parties. Conflict and differences existed but compromise and consensus were the hallmarks of the Swedish system of government and seemed to result in policies which were widely acceptable.

By the 1970s, however, Swedish social democrats were becoming impatient even with the degree of social change that had been accomplished. A high standard of living for most people and social security in its widest sense was not enough. Like those on the left in other countries they began to dream of social engineering on a larger scale. A greater degree of equality and democracy was the aim. It was not enough to make capitalism human;

the system needed fundamental change in order to evolve towards socialism. In education this meant *recurrent* education with the comprehensivisation of the upper secondary school and higher education itself, as well as expanded opportunities for adults. Education was to be about the redistribution of cultural capital (Ball and Larsson, 1989). In social insurance, employers alone were to contribute to their employees' state benefits. Opportunities for parental and educational leave built on the idea of maternity leave were to be created. Laws were passed giving trade unions and their members more rights, greater protection and a bigger say in decision making. Finally the idea of wage-earner funds was proposed. The brainchild of an LO economic adviser, Rudolph Meidner, the wage-earner funds were to require employers to place a proportion of their profits into a fund for the future benefit of their employees, whose trade union representatives would sit on the funds' managing bodies.

The wage-earner funds became an important issue in the general election of 1976. It is always difficult to say what influences voters in a general election but there were those who attributed the social democrats' loss of office after 44 years to this proposal. It is as likely that the electorate were just as worried about other aspects of the social democrats' policies. Sweden's economy had begun to stagnate following the 1973 oil crisis. The public sector already employed a quarter of the workforce. With hindsight one might conclude that the Swedish people were amongst the first to demonstrate what Wilensky had described as the welfare backlash (Wilensky, 1975).

THE BOURGEOIS GOVERNMENTS, 1976–82

But backlash is too strong a word. The social democrats remained the largest party in the Riksdag (Sweden's parliament) and still commanded over 40 per cent of the vote. The new bourgeois government had a slim majority and consisted of the Conservative, Liberal and Centre parties. Not only were there major differences between these three on many social and economic issues, but none of them had really thought through how they would manage a state whose institutions had been so thoroughly dominated by social democratic values and practices. Initially the government found itself continuing to implement reforms which were already in train – though not the wage-earner funds to which the three parties were vehemently opposed. Moreover, faced with an economic situation in which the viability of many firms was under threat, the government proceeded to hand out subsidies and take firms into public ownership on a scale that no social democratic government had ever done (*The Economist*, 1981). Even after a victory in the election of 1979, disunity prevented any real onslaught on the institutions and policies of state welfare. By the time the government had begun to propose cutbacks in social insurance benefits, the public turned again. Whether it was because the electorate had decided it was not ready for the dismantling of the People's Home, or whether people yearned for the return of the natural party of government to replace the squabbling parties of the right, is not easy to say. But, by the time the social democrats were returned to office in 1982, it could be said without much disagreement that the bourgeois government had made matters worse for the economy and had no impact on reducing the size of public sector.

EMERGING CRITICISMS

In the latter half of the 1970s a number of criticisms began to emerge of the Swedish welfare state. Writers such as Furniss and Tilton were still able to use Sweden as an example of a state where a much broader vision of social welfare had been implemented. It went, they claimed, beyond the provision of a minimum level of subsistence as might be found in their own country, the USA, and even beyond the Beveridge social security state of Britain. The Swedish welfare state was built upon a commitment to a high standard of public services for all (Furniss and Tilton, 1977). Neo-Marxists such as Larsson and Sjöström, however disagreed and argued that the social democrats had done little to reduce the inequalities of wealth, income and power that characterised all capitalist societies. Even employment and social welfare policies came under attack for the way in which they directed and controlled the labour force (Larsson and Sjöström 1979). Similar attacks were made upon Swedish corporatism by people like Leo Panitch. They tended to see the way in which the government, business and trade unions managed the organisations of the state as an insidious incorporation of the labour movement by the forces of capital (Panitch, 1981). A slightly different version of the same argument could be found later in Alf Ronnby's *Socialstaten* (1985). Ronnby saw the social democrats and the trade unions and the state apparatus, not as victims of capitalist incorporation but as the key constituents of a vast social technocracy bent on manipulating the very people they were supposed to serve. From a more centrist political position, Dorothy Wilson in 1979 had described a welfare state which had simply gone over the top in providing a degree of security which was likely to impair the incentive both to work and to invest (Wilson, 1979). A more scathing version of this argument suggested that Swedish socialists had milked, and wrecked, a strong free market economy which had been expected to sustain both a bloated bureaucracy and the propaganda activities of trade unions. At the same time they had created a moral malaise in which high rates of crime, divorce, suicide, illegitimate births and alcoholism flourished (Shenfield, 1980).

In an attempt to make sense of these various interpretations the one thing that seemed to concern critics of both the left and the right was the way in which a new class of salaried workers had managed to ensure that they benefited from the Swedish welfare state either as producers or as consumers of welfare. Gould suggested that, to a greater degree than in Britain, the salaried middle class had become a drain on the resources of capital and labour alike (Gould, 1982).

THE RETURN OF THE SOCIAL DEMOCRATS, 1982–88

The gloomier predictions of Sweden's critics seemed to be proved wrong when, in 1982, the SAP was returned to government. Severe economic measures, including a 14 per cent devaluation of the krona brought the economy back on course. The enormous budget deficit bequeathed by the previous government took some years to bring under control but eventually the policies of the Finance Minister, Kjell Olof-Feldt, and the government succeeded even in that. Respectable levels of growth were achieved and yet again the outside world began to marvel at the success of the Swedish model. An article in *The British Economist* (1987) claimed that the Swedish authorities had shown that it was possible to have high public spending and high rates of growth. Martin Linton, in the *Guardian*, under the headline 'By all accounts they should be bust', was full of praise for the way in which social democrats in Sweden had tackled their economic problems without having to sacrifice their commitments to the welfare state and full employment (Linton, 1984a). Linton advised the British Labour Party to take the opportunity of learning from the way the Swedes operated (Linton, 1984b). In a Fabian pamphlet he went further and showed how impressive was the SAP's political organisation. They had more members in the trade unions, in the SAP itself and in its young people's section. More full-time agents worked on the party's behalf and the organisation of the party permeated the lives of ordinary workers in a variety of ways. More importantly, the social democratic state had ensured that the national and local press represented a broad range of political views, unlike in Britain where conservative thinking dominated most newspapers (Linton, 1985).

Far from the public sector being a drain on the economy, it was once again possible to argue that a strong public sector contributed to economic growth. Public spending and tax levels remained high. Even the wage-earner funds were introduced. The election of 1985 was won by the social democrats and the election of 1988. Olsson (1988) was able to argue even in 1988 that the Swedish commitment to the social democratic welfare state was a deep and lasting one. Looking back at developments in the 1980s he described how, with the exception of one major local authority and a number of small experiments, neither privatisation nor growth in private welfare provision had occurred in Sweden on any appreciable scale. On the contrary, a process of decentralisation was taking place in which county councils and the *kommunes* were being given greater responsibilities to run services that before had been controlled by central government. An alternative solution to excessive state bureaucracy had been found in Sweden which required neither massive expenditure cuts nor mass unemployment: decentralisation.

THE INTERNATIONAL CLIMATE

But Olsson's account was premature and over-optimistic. The fundamental difficulties of the Swedish economy and its large public sector had not been dealt with (Heclo and Madsen, 1986). Throughout the 1980s Sweden had devoted over 30 per cent of its gross domestic product to health, social security and social services, while employment in the public sector had grown to account for a third of the labour force (Statistiska Centralbyrån, SCB, 1990). The major problems of inflation, low growth and trade deficits went away from time to time only to return in more serious forms. The strong, centralised trade union movement prevented unemployment being used as an economic weapon. Large companies, with their high labour costs, became uncompetitive and small enterprises found it difficult to survive. But the fact that the whole international climate had changed meant that Sweden could no longer ignore the economic realities which many other advanced capitalist countries had faced by reducing the size of their public sectors and allowing unemployment to grow (Morris, 1988).

Sweden's reputation as the model welfare state had been established when the whole of Europe and America were enjoying the long post-war boom that lasted into the 1960s and early 1970s. Economic growth had made it possible for many countries to finance a growing public sector while individual citizens enjoyed growing personal affluence. This period had been brought to an end by the oil crisis of 1973, after which it was no longer possible to countenance high increases in both private and public spending. Moreover, a new competitor had established itself on the international scene which ignored the prevailing wisdom that a modern industrial economy needed a strong public sector maintained by high levels of taxation in order to finance the health care, education and social security of the whole population and cope with its social problems. Japan had resisted the idea of a European-style welfare state. Its levels of public and social expenditure were low. Its workforce was disciplined. Its population was healthy and educated to an extent which compared well even with Sweden. Moreover, various writers seemed to be agreed that, while social problems existed in Japan, few problems were as disruptive as those found in the West (Vogel, 1979; Pinker, 1986; Rose, 1985; and Rose and Shiratori, 1986).

The Japanese industrial machine suffered only a minor setback after 1973 and continued to make inroads into Western markets while Europe and America were still recovering. The Japanese economy was a very diversified one. While the core workers of large Japanese enterprises had a high degree of job security and company welfare, those on the periphery, working for medium and small-sized companies, were not so fortunate. Health and pension schemes covered most of the population, but some schemes were less generous than others. Moreover, statutory social services did not exist on any large scale. The family, i.e. women, was expected to provide for the needs of the elderly and the handicapped. Even the effective education system was not generously staffed or equipped. But as, if not more, important than any of these factors was the fact that the Japanese at this time had a small percentage of the population above the age of 65.

Faced with a worsening international economic situation and a competitor which was both better organised and not facing the same costs, it is hardly surprising that governments and employers in America and Europe began to take decisions which resulted in their moving closer to the Japanese model and away from the Swedish. Employers began to take more care of their core workers (Murray, 1989). They jettisoned some of their less profitable activities and began to rely more on the vulnerable workforces of their subsidiaries. Governments began to look for ways to reduce their welfare commitments – welfare pluralism, which was Japan's distinguishing feature, became the vogue term. The family, the company, voluntary agencies could provide where the state left a gap. Full employment was a luxury which could no longer be afforded. It was inflationary and gave trade unions too much power to press for higher wages.

Nowhere were these trends acted upon with greater enthusiasm and relish than the UK. Successive governments under the leadership of Margaret Thatcher sought more and more ingenious ways to erode the strength and solidarity of the trade unions, public sector services, nationalised industries and the local authorities. The erosion of state social security benefits, the privatisation of public services and the provision for schools and hospitals to opt out of the state sector, restrictions on local authority spending – all these and more formed part of an overall strategy to roll back the frontiers of the welfare state.

If this could happen to the British welfare state, which Sweden had both influenced and been influenced by, could it happen in Sweden?

RECENT ECONOMIC AND POLITICAL DEVELOPMENTS IN SWEDEN

By 1991 the Swedish economy was in trouble. With inflation having climbed to 11 per cent since 1988 and economic growth the lowest in OECD countries – less than 1 per cent in 1990 and –0.5 per cent predicted for 1991 – fundamental questions were being asked about the Swedish model. OECD figures also showed that the per capita income of Swedes, once second only to that of the US, ranked seventh in the world in 1988 when adjusted for purchasing parity – a little above Japan and only $1, 300 above the UK (*Dagens Nyheter*, DN, 16 November 1990).

Understandably these trends had made for difficulties in labour relations. Manual workers felt that their real incomes had not grown; those in the public sector expected their incomes to grow at the same rate as those in the private sector. This in turn presented difficulties, given that the public sector now employed one-third of the country's workforce. The wage solidarity policy no longer seemed to function and the gap between SAF and LO in the annual pay negotiations was getting wider. Without agreements to keep pay levels down, the government was being forced into taking measures which allowed unemployment to increase. In the latter part of the 1980s the rate had remained below 2 per cent, but it rose to 2.5 per cent towards the end of 1990. There was a growing consensus that unemployment must be allowed to grow further, with talk of a rate of 5 per cent and more.

A Swedish government faced with increased unemployment inevitably talked of measures to alleviate the problem, particularly for young people for whom unemployment was already high (7 per cent for 16–19 year olds and over 4 per cent for those between 20 and 24; DN, 13 February 1991). If those percentages were to grow then even more young people would be on government training and work experience schemes. Yet it was clear from studies done of the early 1980s, when youth unemployment had been 11 per cent, that these measures were far from unproblematic. As in the UK there had been resentment amongst the young that there were no jobs for them, only government palliatives (Hartmann, 1987); there had been conflict between employers and trade unions about whether 'trainees' should receive an allowance or the rate for the job; and the labour market service had been concerned that unemployed youngsters on local authority schemes should be made to devote time to searching for real jobs. Those who had refused offers of places on schemes had had their benefit withdrawn to discourage dependency (Jonzon and Wise, 1989). It was just this kind of polarisation that the Swedish system had always hoped to avoid.

If there was a parallel between the conflicts and resentments created by growing unemployment in Sweden and the UK, parallels also existed in terms of anxieties about the size of the public sector and the high taxation required to finance it. In one opinion poll 96 per cent of those asked considered that Swedish society was headed in the wrong direction, 84 per cent that the public sector was ineffective, 58 per cent wanted taxes reduced and twice as many thought the policies of the bourgeois parties would be more likely to lead to increased investment in the economy than would the policies of the socialists (DN, 14 December 1990). This political climate was reflected in opinion polls about voting intentions. In May 1989 support for the SAP had dipped just below 40 per cent and the Conservative Party had had only 18.8 per cent. For most of 1990 the SAP had hovered just above 30 per cent. By April 1991, SAP support stood at 28 per cent with the Conservatives at 24.4 per cent, less than four points behind. Although support for the Centre and Liberal parties had declined, KDS, a party of conservative Christian Democrats, had risen to nearly 7 per cent, while both the erstwhile Communist Party (now the Left Party) and the Environment Party had sunk to 4 per cent. Even more serious, bearing in mind the split in the British Labour Party in the early 1980s, was the emergence of the populist New Democracy Party, which then had 12 per cent of the electorate behind it. While the support for the smaller parties may have been volatile, the fall of SAP and the rise of the Conservatives seemed more constant. With the elections about to take place in September 1991 it was hard to imagine that the SAP could reverse the adverse trend significantly.

Not that the government hadn't tried to do so. Attempts had been made to introduce austerity measures and tax reforms with varying degrees of success. Austerity measures had had to be introduced every few months since the elections in September 1988. But the problem for the minority social democrats was that the communists would not support such measures and the unions vociferously opposed them. In consequence the government had had to rely on support from one or more of the bourgeois parties, which then sought to gain policy concessions of their own in exchange. In 1989, a rise in VAT had been introduced only with the last minute support of the Centre Party. In February 1990, Kjell Olof-Feldt had been forced to resign because of pressure from LO when, as Finance Minister, he had tried to introduce a wage and price freeze plus a veto on strikes. On that occasion the Liberal Party had come to the government's rescue and a revised package including a ceiling on the expenditure of local *kommunes* had been introduced.

By October of the same year, another economic crisis had required support for a range of measures. The government had wanted to make cuts of 10 billion kronor in the social insurance budget. This had involved proposals to reduce sickness benefit and for the introduction of waiting days. Other ministries had also been expected to make cuts and a three-year programme to slim central government administration by 10 per cent had been proposed (DN, 23 and 27 October 1990). LO had objected to reductions in sickness insurance and had opposed any attempt to reform the work injury insurance scheme. Again much negotiation with the bourgeois parties had been necessary. Yet even in the midst of compromises and cutbacks the government had raised the basic child allowance by 34 per cent (from 6,720 kronor per child per year to 9,000; 10 kronor equal approximately £1) and the allowances for the fourth and subsequent children! An even more surprising part of the same package of measures had been the announcement that the government would be seeking membership of the European Community. Membership of the EC had been resisted for many years by the social democrats, not merely in the interests of preserving sovereignty in domestic policy, but also because it was thought that closer European cooperation would compromise Swedish foreign policy and neutrality. It took the force of overriding economic imperatives to effect this change of position (though the adjustment was made easier by developments in Eastern Europe, since these were thought likely to change the cold war politics of NATO).

Earlier in the year the government had been able to get support for major tax reforms with less difficulty. Although income tax in Sweden had long had a reputation for being highly progressive with high marginal rates of tax, it had not been so well known that a wide range of tax allowances had made the system extremely complex. For many years the tax system had been criticised for impairing the incentive to work and invest and of promoting a sizeable black market in the economy. Södersten (1990) had explained how internal pressures to reduce marginal rates and allowances had combined with international influences to force changes in policy. He had argued that many of Sweden's international competitors had already introduced taxation reforms and that Swedish multinationals were beginning to move 'their top executives and their central management functions abroad'. These factors and moves towards greater European integration had made reform inevitable. The reforms enacted in June 1990 had come into force in January 1991. Those earning under 170,000 kronor a year were to pay a local income tax only of 30 per cent, while those earning in excess of 170,000 kronor were to pay the same local tax and an additional 20 per cent to central government revenues. Together with the reduction and abolition of certain allowances and an increase in VAT, lower marginal rates and simplification had been achieved at a stroke.

While the tax reform had been a welcome one which had had broad support in Swedish society, the complaint of many Swedes – in particular the supporters of the Conservative and the Liberal parties – was that the overall tax burden remained too high. The social democrats had simplified the system and they had reduced marginal tax rates; but the same amount of tax revenue was still being taken out of the economy. For that reason, the major political parties were beginning to compete with each other in terms of promises of tax reductions after the forthcoming general election.

RECENT SOCIAL POLICY DEVELOPMENTS

Without cuts in public expenditure, the Swedish welfare state faced formidable problems. The growing proportion of elderly people in the population continued to have repercussions for pensions, health care and social services. The promise by the government to provide child care for all who needed it had been complicated by the recent sharp increase in the birth rate. Rising unemployment was costly, given the high standards of Swedish benefit schemes. Sickness benefit costs and the numbers receiving disability pensions had also been increasing. All of these developments meant that ways had to be found to prioritise the use of existing resources, thus forcing the welfare authorities down exactly the same path as many other West European countries.

Decentralisation was creating problems for the *kommunes*. They could not increase their tax rates, and central government was cutting state grants. At the same time extra responsibilities were coming their way. All things being equal the new responsibilities would have been welcome, but without extra resources it was difficult to see how they would be able to cope with the kommunalisation of care for the elderly and of schools. Neither of those measures were yet in place but when they were they would mean a transfer of responsibilities for medical services from the county council health care authorities and a transfer from central government of responsibilities for education. In the prevailing economic climate it was not difficult to foresee the arguments about resource transfers that would be likely to result.

Hospitals were having to rationalise and prioritise in order to cope with lengthy waiting lists, which varied from a few months to in excess of two years for certain operations (*Svenska Dagbladet*, SvD, 1989c). The Diagnosis Related Groups (DRG) system borrowed from the USA was beginning to have an impact. DRG enabled hospitals to cost operations and types of treatment with the aim of improving management, planning and evaluation. Units within hospitals were setting themselves up as private entities, selling their services to other departments, hospitals and areas. There were claims in Lund that such changes resulted in more operations, fewer queues and lower costs (SvD, 1989d). Others, like doctors in Västerås, insisted the reforms were inefficient (SvD, 1989f). Doctors in Huddinge had complained of nurse shortages, resource shortages and the consequent need to ration care (SvD, 1989e, f). Pay differentials for nurses were increasing as county councils found that they could not all afford to pay the same rates (SvD, 1989b).

While the government merely claimed that more efficiency was needed rather than more resources, the Conservative and the Liberal parties insisted that competition from an expanded private sector was required. While doctors complained of shortages, private consultants claimed that 50 per cent of the administrators in Stockholm County's health service were surplus to requirements. Savings were being sought by closing departments up and down the country. Health authorities were laying off workers, particularly the temporary ones who made up 27 per cent of the workforce. Belatedly, the use of generic drugs was being considered in an effort to make savings (DN, 11 June 1990). From January 1991 the charge for a visit to a doctor was to go up 66 per cent from 60 to 100 kronor.

The difficulties faced by local *kommunes* in Sweden has already been referred to. Their social service departments now had the responsibility for much of the care of the elderly which had previously been discharged by the county councils. Yet there were real transitional problems, given that long-stay institutions had already been closed in anticipation of the build-up of community care resources to cope with elderly people locally. Again, as far as child care was concerned, the commitment to provide day care for all those that needed it by 1991 was proving very difficult and had not been helped by the economic crisis. In the face of continuing waiting lists, some day care establishments were reducing their intakes. Alternatives were also being sought. Parents' cooperatives had been set up in Malmö (DN, 28 June 1990). More and more private companies were wanting to set up their own crèches (SvD, 21 September 1989).

Pressures existed in the area of compulsory care both for children and for adult substance misusers. On the one hand the annual budget for such care was considerable – 950 million kronor in 1990 (DN, 22 December 1990). On the other hand there were considered to be many children in need who were simply not being found places (DN, 12 December 1990). There was also concern about the growing costs of means-tested social assistance – also administered by the *kommunes*' social services departments. There had been a sharp increase in the numbers on social assistance and hence in its total cost after the introduction of the liberalising Social Services Act of 1982, though since 1986 the costs had been fairly steady. The first six months of 1990 suggested, however, that record levels might be reached by the end of that year, with a possible increase in real terms of 20 per cent on the previous year's costs (DN, 2 November 1990).

Meanwhile the same rising costs had been causing problems for the administrative board for social insurance (SFV). Between 1987 and 1988 the costs of sickness benefit had risen by 35 per cent, or 8 billion kronor, only a quarter of which increase had been due to inflation. The rest had been largely due to a reform implemented in 1987 and an increase in the number of days for which benefit had been claimed (SvD, 1989a). In addition, the numbers of people on disability pensions had risen from 250,000 in 1984 to 300,000 in 1988 (SCB, 1986 and 1990). These increases had prompted a great deal of concern. A major debate had taken place about the role of rehabilitation in relation to long-term sickness benefit and disability pensions, since it was felt that many of those on benefit could work, given the right sort of help. But inevitably this sort of proposal raised fears about the sick and injured being forced back to work against their will.

After the crisis proposals of October 1990 it was finally agreed, with the support of the Centre and Conservative parties, that sickness benefit would be reduced to 65 per cent of earnings for the first three days, 80 per cent for 3 – 90 days and 90 per cent thereafter, with employers responsible for paying 10 per cent of benefit. Parental leave for looking after sick children was also reduced to 80 per cent of pay for the first 14 days (DN, 8 December 1990).

Less easy to reduce were pensions for the elderly. It had been calculated that, with an annual growth rate in GDP of 2 per cent, contributions to the state earnings-related pension scheme (ATP) would remain at a steady 20 per cent of employers' wage costs; a growth rate of 1 per cent would result in contributions of almost 40 per cent by 2035, while nil growth would mean contributions of over 50 per cent (Ståhlberg, 1990). All of which was leading to proposals to reduce the cost: by linking pension increases to wages instead of prices, by not increasing the ceiling beyond which ATP is not paid and/or by increasing the maximum number of years of contributions necessary to draw full benefit from 30 to 40. Ståhlberg (1990) had even proposed a run down of the present pay-as-you-go system and its replacement by funded occupational pensions. Subsequently, the government had proposed to rescue the finances of ATP by abandoning the wage-earner funds and transferring their resources to the state earnings-related pension scheme – thus causing considerable annoyance to the parties of the right (DN, 4 February 1991).

As the social democrats were forced by a variety of circumstances to water down or abandon some of their principal programmes, it also became clear that in important respects social policy developments in the previous 20 years had failed to achieve their anticipated goals. A set of essays on Swedish education showed that, while educational provision had expanded for all groups in society, little impact had been made upon class and gender inequalities. Young women were still much more likely to 'choose' non-technical subjects at school and finish up in the 'caring lines' at university. As a result women predominated in the public sector of the economy while men predominated in the private sector. Nor had there been much change in the previous 20 years in the proportions of children from manual worker backgrounds compared with those from higher occupational groups going into academic lines in the *gymnasieskolor* (upper secondary schools) which prepared students for university. A number of contributors to these essays also agreed that little more than lip-service had been paid in the education system to the aims of greater democracy and the redistribution of cultural power in the previous decade (Ball and Larsson, 1989). The radical aims of the early 1970s had been replaced by economic priorities. The post-1968 participatory rationale for greater opportunities for young people, women and adults generally, had succumbed in the 1980s to the requirements of the labour market.

Research published by the Social Medicine Institute in Stockholm had shown that, whereas death rates for manual workers and white-collar workers had been almost identical in the early 1960s, since that time the death rates for the former had increased while for the latter they had decreased by 25 per cent (DN, 30 November 1990). An official report into children's mental health had shown that, although differences between socioeconomic groups had narrowed during the 1950s, the children of manual workers were now four to five times more likely to have serious social and mental problems than those from other socioeconomic groups (DN, 21 February 1991). A similar pattern held true for children's heights. In 1960 there had been hardly any difference between the heights of 7-year-old children with parents in manual as compared with non-manual work, but since then the differences had increased (DN, 13 March 1991).

A parallel development had been observed by Bo Södersten who had argued that the tax advantages for housing loans enjoyed by the middle mass of the population in the 1970s and 1980s, had, because of inflation, created wide economic differences between those who owned their own houses and those who did not. He put it graphically by suggesting that, whereas the middle class had been able to manipulate tax allowances to their considerable advantage, the working class could manipulate only sickness benefits through days off work (Södersten, 1990).

CONCLUSION

By 1991, the middle way had become a cul-de-sac. It was being eroded under the pressures created by full employment and a large public sector in a hostile economic environment. Sweden had been forced by circumstances to seek to join the European Community. In doing so, and in recognising the international pressures which beset the country, unemployment was being allowed to rise and welfare benefits were being reduced. Cuts in public services would leave female employees particularly vulnerable.

Increasingly, public services were being forced to become more efficient, more accountable and to manage with fewer resources. Moreover, alternative sources of provision were becoming attractive in a system once dominated by the state.

How Swedish society would cope with these changes was difficult to predict. On the one hand, trade unions and public sector employees had been so used to exerting pressure on government that it might prove difficult, even for a more coherent and more purposeful bourgeois coalition, to bring about the changes that it would like to see. It was unlikely that the left would collapse as it had in the UK or that a bourgeois – or any other – coalition would be possessed of the same radical, free market intent as British governments in the 1980s. The result of any impasse might prove very damaging to the competitiveness of the Swedish economy in the long term.

On the other hand, as Pempel (1990) had pointed out, Sweden, like Japan, had been extremely successful at managing capitalism in the past. Moreover, with the exception of the Conservatives, the bourgeois parties in Sweden were not ideologically hostile to state welfare, only to what they saw as its excesses. It might yet turn out that the traditions of consensus and compromise in Swedish politics would enable whatever coalition emerged in the autumn of 1991 to restore strength to the economy and make the public sector slimmer and more efficient, without the ideological destructiveness that had accompanied Thatcherism in Britain. It was important to remember that the Swedish welfare state had been built on a large scale and upon firm, deep-rooted foundations. It might be able to survive a lot more trimming than most and come through the experience the stronger for it.

But the lesson was being learnt the hard way. It was simply not possible for a capitalist country in an internationally competitive economy to allow its public sector to outstrip all others.

POSTSCRIPT POST SEPTEMBER 1991

This chapter was first drafted in May 1991. Only in the closing stages of revision has it been possible to take into account subsequent events leading up to and including the election on 15th September and the formation of a new government.

As far as social policy is concerned, many of the trends already observed continue. Cuts in the administration of education have led to over two-thirds of personnel losing their jobs. Serious reductions have also been seen in local education budgets, with home language tuition for immigrant children and adult education taking the brunt. Health tests at school, which had been compulsory for many years, have become voluntary, while new evidence suggests that class inequalities in children's health and diet are increasing.

Community care continues to present problems, with the *kommunes* complaining that mental hospitals are discharging difficult patients who cannot cope in the community. There have also been worries that the closing of old people's homes was premature. Research from SCB showed that the costs of the home help service and of social assistance had both doubled in the 1980s. Meanwhile the National Board for Social Affairs has complained that many *kommunes* were paying social assistance at rates lower than those recommended.

The sickness benefit reforms seemed to have a rapid effect. The numbers claiming benefit by July were down by over 25 per cent. Research by SCB and the Social Insurance Board suggested that it was the lowest paid who were worst hit by the reforms. Whereas it was claimed that parental insurance was much more likely to be used by middle class parents, who found it easier to get time off work.

It has also become clear that, not only had the low paid been worse hit by the reforms in taxation, but their relative position in terms of income had deteriorated in the 1980s. The latter was a serious admission by LO which had prided itself on a continued policy of wage solidarity aimed at reducing income differentials. It is also reported that union membership has been declining, with the result that the unionisation levels of manual and non-manual unions are now similar.

If the power and significance of trade unions seem to be on the wane, the employers' federation, SAF, has decided that it no longer wishes to play a role in the state's corporatist machinery. It clearly feels that its ability to represent its members' interests has been compromised by the constant negotiations involved in participation on national and local administrative boards. This is ironic when one considers that it was so often those on the left who had levelled the charge of 'incorporation' and 'betrayal' at trade union involvement in the machinery of the capitalist state.

Support for the public sector amongst voters has also declined. In 1986 the proportion of those who wished to see a reduced public sector was 37 per cent with 32 per cent wishing to see an expansion. Four years later those proportions had respectively become 56 per cent and 18 per cent. Opinion polls right up to July reflected this feeling by the low level of support for the social democrats.

The final months of the election campaign were characterised by arguments about the role of New Democracy in any bourgeois coalition and by disagreements over a number of policy issues within the established bourgeois parties. New Democracy, which for some months had enjoyed about 10 per cent support in the polls, had emerged as a populist base for those discontented with the traditional party system. It clearly had policies which would adversely affect immigrants, refugees and women. So much so that both the Liberal Party and the Centre Party stated very clearly that they could not be part of any coalition which included New Democrats.

Meanwhile, a number of significant disagreements emerged amongst the bourgeois parties. They could not even say categorically which of the party leaders was the prime minister-elect. However, the Liberal and the Conservative parties did produce a joint policy document entitled, 'A New Start for Sweden' (*Ny Start för Sverige*, 1991). It stated that the two parties were agreed that they should promote a market economy, competition and individual choice; that they would reduce taxes, promote growth and restore price stability in order to halt stagnation. The details set out a clear neo-liberal choice for the electorate, but it was not one accepted by the Centre Party. Nor was the Centre Party entirely happy about the commitment shared by the other major parties about entry into Europe or about a future reliance on nuclear energy (an issue which had caused serious splits in the bourgeois bloc during the 1976–82 period). Serious divisions also arose over child care. While all distanced themselves from the social democratic policy of state-provided care for all who needed it, there was disagreement about what to put in its place and when. A monthly care allowance was proposed by the conservatives, the Centre Party and the christian democrats, but they disagreed on the amount and the timing of the reform. The liberals wanted a compromise which lay somewhere between their bourgeois partners and the social democrats – arguing for a lump sum for the parent(s) at the birth of a child and a commitment to a degree of state care. By September, it could hardly be said that the bourgeois bloc was presenting a coherent image to the electorate.

The result, in the end, was a strange one, as can be seen from Table 8.1. The Social Democrats received almost 38 per cent of the vote and the Left Party 4.5 per cent. Although not as bad as had been expected some months previously, the socialist bloc had suffered a clear reversal – down 7 per cent on 1988. If the support for New Democracy was added to that of the four traditional bourgeois parties, then the centre–right bloc had 53 per cent of the vote. It could be said that not only had the Swedish electorate moved away from the left, but it had also moved away from the centre – since both the Centre and the Liberal parties had lost ground (each having lost around 3 per cent support since 1988).

But while the right could claim an overall victory, it was a flawed one. The conservatives improved their performance by only 3.6 per cent. They still remained small in comparison with many of their European counterparts. Much of the support lost by the left and the centre had gone to the christian democrats and New Democracy. So when the Speaker in the Riksdag asked Carl Bildt, the Conservative leader, to form a government, the task was not an easy one. The Liberal and the Centre parties had made it clear

Table 8.1   Swedish Election Results, September 1991

Party	Votes	(%) Change since 1988	No. of seats
Conservatives	21.9	+3.6	80
Liberals	9.1	−3.1	33
Centre	8.5	−2.8	31
Christian Democrats	7.1	+4.2	26
New Democracy	6.7	−	25
Environment Party	3.4	−2.1	− [a]
Social Democrats	37.6	−5.6	138
Left Party	4.5	−1.3	16
			349

Note: [a] Parties have to achieve a minimum of 4% of the vote to obtain seats in the Riksdag.

that they would not share power with New Democracy. A majority government was therefore impossible. That left Bildt with the choice of going for a minority government based on four, three or even two parties. The larger the number of parties the greater parliamentary support he would have, the smaller the number of parties the more cohesive his government would be. The outcome was a four-party centre–right coalition excluding New Democracy. The irony is that, were Bildt's government to fail, then the Social Democrats, the Centre Party and the Liberal Party could in fact form a majority centre–left government.

Other important features of the election worth noting were, firstly, that, because local government elections in Sweden are held at the same time as general elections, the results, not surprisingly, were similar to the national ones. There was therefore likely to be a clear rightward shift in social policy at both the national and local levels. Secondly, the number of women in the Riksdag had fallen from 132 to 100, a reflection of the fact that the more right-wing parties had fewer women candidates than those on the left. Thirdly, 75 per cent of first-time voters had voted for the centre–right parties as a whole, 35 per cent of them for the Conservatives and only 20 per cent for the social democrats. It was perhaps ominous that these latter percentages were the reverse of the national picture.

NOTES

1   The main body of this paper was written in advance of the elections of September 1991, but a post-election postscript appears at the end.

REFERENCES

Ball, S. and Larsson, S. (1989) *The Struggle for Democratic Education*, Lewes, Sussex: Falmer.

Childs, M. (1936) *The Middle Way*, New Haven, Conn.: Yale University Press.

DN [Dagens Nyheter]:
11 June 1990, 'Billigare läkemedel löser vårdkrisen'
28 June 1990, 'Bostadsbolag barnskötare'
23 October 1990, 'Sociala utgifter bantas hårt'
27 October 1990, 'Så här slår krispaketet'
2 November 1990, 'Sociala bidragen ökar kraftigt'
16 November 1990, 'Svårt för Sverige hävda sig'
30 November 1990, 'Arbetare dör yngre'
8 December 1990, 'Lägre sjukpenning'
12 December 1990, 'Ungdom i kris helt utan vård'
14 December 1990, '86 procent vill ha systemskifte'
22 December 1990, 'Öronmärkt bidrag'
4 February 1991, 'Löntagarfonderna skrotas'
13 February 1991, 'Fler unga utan Jobb'
21 February 1991, 'Barns hälsa en klassfråga'
13 March 1991, 'Klassskillnader tillbaka'

Economist, The (1981) 'Swedish industry's thin upper crust', 4 April.

—— (1987) 'The non-conformist state', 7 March.

Furniss, N. and Tilton, T. (1977) *The Case for the welfare state*, Bloomington: Indiana University Press.

Gould, A. (1982) 'The salaried middle class and the welfare state in Sweden and Japan', in *Policy and Politics* 10(4).

Hartmann, J. (1987) 'New forms of youth participation and work' in *Sweden International Social Science Journal* 37(106).

Heclo, H. and Madsen, M. (1986) *Policy and Politics in Sweden*, Philadelphia: Temple University Press.

Jonzon, B. and Wise, L.R. (1989) 'Getting young people to work', *International Labour Review* 128(3).

Larsson, S. and Sjöström, K. (1979) 'The welfare state myth in class society' in J. Fry, *The Limits of the welfare state*, Aldershot: Saxon House.

Linton, M. (1984a) 'By all accounts they should be bust', *Guardian* 9 October.

—— (1984b) 'How Labour could go its own Swede way', *Guardian*, September.

—— (1985) *The Swedish Road to Socialism*, London: Fabian Society.

Morris, R.(ed.) *Testing the Limits of Social Welfare*, London: Brandeis University Press.

Murray, R. (1989) 'Fordism and Post-Fordism' in J. Hall and M. Jacques, *New Times*, London: Lawrence & Wishart.

Ny Start för Sverige (1991) Stockholm: Moderaterna and Folkpartiet Liberalerna.

Olsson, S. (1988) 'Decentralisation and privatisation: strategies against a welfare backlash in Sweden', in R. Morris (ed.) *Testing the Limits of Social Welfare*, London: Brandeis University Press.

Panitch, L. (1981) 'Trade unions and the corporatist state', *New Left Review*, no. 125.

Pempel, T.J. (1990) 'Japan and Sweden: polarities of responsible capitalism', in D. Rustow and K. Erickson (eds) *Comparative Political Dynamics*, New York: Harper & Row.

Pinker, R. (1986) 'Social welfare in Japan and Britain', in E. Oyen *Comparing welfare states and Their Futures*, Aldershot: Gower.

Ronnby, A. (1985) *Socialstaten*, Lund: Studentlitteratur.

Rose, R. (1985) 'Welfare: the lesson from Japan', *New Society*, 28 June.

Rose, R. and Shiratori, R. (eds) (1986) *Welfare state: East and West*, Oxford: Oxford University Press.

Shenfield, A. (1980) *The Failure of Socialism*, Washington DC: Heritage Foundation.

Södersten, B. (1990) 'The Swedish tax reform', *Current Sweden*, no. 375.

SCB (1986) Statistisk Årsbok Stockholm: Statistika Centralbyrån.

—— (1990) Statistisk Årsbok Stockholm: Statistika Centralbyrån.

Ståhlberg, A.C. (1990) 'Lessons from the Swedish pension system' in D. Wilson (ed.) *The Objectives of the welfare state*, Oxford: Blackwell.

SvD [Svenska Dagbladet]:
  31 May 1989a, 'Sjukförsäkringen blev 35 procent dyrare i fjol',
  6 August 1989b, 'Sjöterskors löneskillnader växer',
  6 August 1989c, 'Färre operationer på Karolinska',
  8 August 1989d, 'Effektiva kirurger i Lund skapar hjärtkön med hälften',
  28 August 1989e, 'Läkare tvingas sålla patienter',
  30 August 1989f, 'Huddinge sjukhus är inte något sjunkande skepp',
  21 September 1989g, 'Dagis på arbetsplatsen sista utvägen',

Tomasson, R. (1970) *Sweden: Prototype of Modern Society*, New York: Random House.

Vogel, E. (1979) *Japan as Number One*, Cambridge, Mass.: Harvard University Press.

Wilensky, H. (1975) *The Welfare State and Equality: Structural and Ideological Roots of Public Expenditures*, Berkeley and Los Angeles: University of California Press.

Wilson, D. (1979) *The welfare state in Sweden*, London: Heinemann.

9 Developments in East European social policy

Bob Deacon

INTRODUCTION

This chapter is divided into four parts. First, I shall summarise the main characteristics of the system of social welfare that existed across Eastern Europe and in the Soviet Union before the reforms and revolutions of 1989 and indicate the social policy problems bequeathed by 'communism' to the successor regimes. Then, I shall summarise the main trends in social policy that have emerged since the collapse of the old regimes in 1989. Here we will notice the extent of commonality across the several countries of Eastern Europe and focus on the common issues for social policy in this period of transition and also notice beginnings of the diversification of development. Lastly, I shall locate the emergent diversification of social policy regime types within the comparative social policy literature that offers typologies of Western welfare states. I shall ask whether the East is merely copying the West or whether new types of post-communist welfare regimes are emerging.

SOCIAL POLICY BEFORE THE COLLAPSE OF COMMUNISM: A BALANCE SHEET

Had we been present in 1989 and able to stop the clock of the revolutions of Eastern Europe or present in 1991 and able to intervene in the collapse of Soviet communism, what, as analysts of capitalist welfare states, might we have wished to preserve? For some internal critics of the old regime the answer was simple: very little. Julia Szalai stated in 1989 before the end of 'communism' in Hungary (Deacon and Szalai, 1990: 92):

> What social policy gives its subjects are the many irritating, humiliating and painful experiences of unfairness, defencelessness and chronic shortage. Social policy has come to be associated with widely unsatisfied needs, with unacceptable bureaucratic regulations, with haphazard provision of services at more and more unacceptable levels.

Table 9.1 A system of welfare across Eastern Europe and the Soviet Union

Advantages	Disadvantages
Job security for many	Inadequate or absent unemployment pay
Workers' wages high percentage of average wages	Hidden privileges of party/state bureaucrats
Free health services (but oiled with bribes and gifts)	Underdevelopment of preventative approach to health. High mortality/ morbidity rates
Three-year childcare grants for working women and the right to return to work (especially in the GDR and Hungary)	Obligation upon women to work and care. Sexist division of labour
Highly subsidised flats	Maldistribution of flats so better off live in most heavily subsidised
State-organised social security pension and sick pay system	No index-linking of benefits and heavily work record regulated. Totally inadequate back-up social aid
State party/workplace paternalism	Total absence of rights to articulate social needs autonomously from below

On the other hand, Western social policy analysts (Arato and Feher, 1989) have drawn attention to the ways in which heavily subsidised foods and rents, full employment, the relatively high (as a percentage of average) wages of workers, the provision of free or cheap health, education and cultural services represented a type of welfare contract between the party-state apparatus and the people which was marred only by its inefficiency and the hidden privileges of the nomenklatura. In Table 9.1 we try to draw up a balance sheet of positive and negative features of the pre-1989 system. Additionally, Table 9.2 provides some summary social data for the 1980's: a snapshot of the later days of bureaucratic state collectivism compared with similar data for countries within the OECD.

The right to work was generally enshrined in the constitution. A place of work was indeed available for the vast majority of the population, both men and women. Often, however, this was a way of hiding unemployment. Little productive work actually took place in many workplaces. The regimes pretended to pay such workers and the workers pretended to work. In many countries, most notably Hungary but the practice existed elsewhere, wages from official workplaces were so low that an adequate standard of living could be secured only by taking a second or even third job in the unofficial

Table 9.2 Some social indicators at the end of bureaucratic state collectivism

Indicator	Soviet Union	Bulgaria	Czech-oslovakia	German Democratic Republic	Hungary	Poland	Romania	OECD
Population (in millions)	286.4	9.0	15.6	16.6	10.6	38.0	23.0	824.8
GDP per capita (US dollars)	5,552	5,633	7,603	9,361	6,491	5,453	4,117	14,637
Cars per 1,000 inhabitants	50	127	182	206	153	74	11	385
Life expectancy (average m/f)	70	72	71	73	70	72	70	76
Infant mortality per 1,000 live births (0–1 year)	27.3	–	29.4	–	33.8	28.8	–	61.0
Workers with secondary education (%)	25	14	13	8	16	16	24	8

Source: *World Development Report 1990*, World Book; *European Community and its Eastern Neighbours*, European Commission, Office of Official Publications.

Note: all data for 1988 except cars per population, which is 1987.

economy which was often dependent on the utilisation of resources formally belonging to the official place of work. For those who lost their job for political and other reasons, no system of insurance benefits existed. For those regarded variously as work-shy or rejecting of the socialist work ethic little was provided. Gypsy minorities lived on the margins of these societies as a reserve army of labour with no rights and entitlements by virtue of citizenship.

The relatively high (as a percentage of average) wages of sections of the working class – miners, transport workers, construction workers – could be seen as one of the reasons for these societies to be regarded, in a very limited sense, as workers' states. Certainly the relatively privileged position of miners compared with that of middle-ranking professionals (doctors and teachers) was a source of much resentment amongst the latter. This feature, however, co-existed with the hidden privileges of much of the party-state apparatus who had access to hidden incomes and welfare services. It was the 'unjustly' deserved privileges that became a source of much anger, especially in the GDR, during the revolutions of 1989.

Many services, including medical care services, were provided free at the point of use. There was often an extensive system of work-based medical provision. The number of doctors and hospital beds was higher than in comparable West European countries. The service provided was, however, totally inefficient, undercapitalised and often lacking in basic equipment. Only in specialist enclaves did excellence exist. While often professing a prophylactic approach to health, the governments of Eastern Europe and the Soviet Union systematically injured the health of their populations by requiring work in health-damaging environments, by polluting the earth and atmosphere, and by presiding over a social system that encouraged alcoholism, an unhealthy diet, and suicide. The mortality rates for Eastern Europe compare very unfavourably with those of comparable capitalist societies and throughout the 1960s and 1970s and most of the 1980s these were worsening. Recent data from the Soviet Union (Mezentseva and Rimachevskaya, 1990) suggest improvements following in the wake of the anti-alcohol campaign. Only in the Central Asian republics of the Soviet Union did health indicators compare favourably with neighbouring and equivalent Iran and Turkey. McAuley (1991) reported life expectancy for males and females in Central Asia in 1979/80 as 63.2 and 69.8, compared with figures of 55.8 and 55.0 for Iran and 60.0 and 63.3 for Turkey. Soviet socialist imperialism does seem to have had an improving impact on aspects of the quality of life of its southern colonial republics but this, of course, at the expense of the autonomous right of the republics to self-determination.

Benefits and services provided to ease the situation of working women were quite extensive in many of the East European countries. The three-year child care grant in Hungary and comparable benefits in the GDR had attracted the approval of comparative analysts. An extensive system of creche and kindergarten services complemented the cash benefits. Often, except in Romania, abortion legislation was liberal. The other side of the coin was the obligation upon women to work and be carers, the unreconstructed division of labour in the home between men and women, the poor quality of many of the communal services and the lack of user involvement in them. Abortion was often the most available form of contraception.

Housing was cheap. Rents were a very small proportion of income. The right to a place to live was a policy actively being implemented by many East European governments. The inefficiency of the house-building industry and the lack of priority given to it in earlier years had led, however, to extensive shortages. Twenty-year waiting lists were not uncommon. Enforced three-generation and post-divorce communalism was common. Even enforced communal kitchens and bathrooms, a distorted legacy of the idealised communalism of the early Bolsheviks, were common. Gypsy houses were built recently by councils with no running water, no sewerage, no pavements and no lighting. The better flats often came to be allocated to the state-party apparatus. The redistributors benefited from the redistribution. Recent evidence from the Soviet Union (Zaslavskaya 1990) suggested house building was becoming a major priority in the early *perestroika* days.

Certainly the system of social security against the risks of sickness and old age was well developed and often provided for benefits that, initially, were a high proportion of wages. However, the absence of inflation proofing turned these benefits, over time, into gifts of the state that might or might not be uprated periodically. There was a heavily work-related element in the benefits system. Retirement could, however, take place at a relatively young age. The other side of the coin of the social security systems was the paternalistic, parsimonious and cash-limited social aid system administered by local authorities. For those falling outside the insured categories of risk, provision was totally inadequate. Allocation according to work record rather than need led to unmet and extensive need among widows, the young, the disabled, single parents, alcoholics and others outcast by the society.

The state, often through the agency of the workplace or trade union did indeed exercise a paternalistic concern for those in established workplaces with good work records. Holiday homes, sanatoria, housing and other benefits came with the job. The obverse of this system was the virtual absence of any right or facility to articulate welfare needs from below, either in the workplace or outside it. Prior to 1989, organisations such as the Society for the Protection of the Poor (SZETA) in Hungary were outlawed and subject to police harassment.

We arrive at the paradox that, if they existed in the context of the democratic pluralist politics of the capitalist economies of Western Europe, some of the social policies of the old Eastern Europe (child care grants and the guarantee of work for mothers and fathers, liberal abortion legislation, subsidised housing, benefit levels set at a high percentage of average earnings) would be heralded by many as the progressive achievements of the social democratic regulation of market capitalism; whereas within Eastern Europe they were perceived as part and parcel of the totalitarian state project of forcing work out of reluctant citizens for purposes which seemed to benefit only the privileged party state apparatus.

We are also faced with the conclusion that the positive (from the Western critics standpoint) features of East European social policy – its egalitarianism for example – sit side by side with an underdeveloped and inefficient economy. The East European experience does underline the point that a balance of advantages has to be struck between economic efficiency and distributive justice. We are reminded of Kornai's (1986: 124) conclusion that:

> It is impossible to create a closed and consistent socio-economic normative theory which would assert, without contradiction, a political-ethical value system and would at the same time provide for the efficiency of the economy ... What compromises are brought about between the different normative principles by the social forces of different systems ... [is a scientific question].

The balance that had been struck historically in Eastern Europe and the Soviet Union had favoured an egalitarianism of underdevelopment. This understanding prompted, of course, Gorbachev in the very early days of *perestroika* to pronounce against crude egalitarianism and social levelling.

> Equalising attitudes crop up from time to time even today. Some citizens understood the call for social justice as 'equalising everyone'. . . . On this point we want to be perfectly clear: socialism has nothing to do with equalising. Socialism has a different criterion for distributing social benefits 'From each according to his ability, to each according to his work'.
>
> (Gorbachev, 1987: 100)

The inefficiency of the economy which reduced the resources available to fund social measures also, of course, operated within the social services so that those free services, such as health, were themselves inadequate by Western standards.

The second general conclusion is that the system of welfare, such as it was, had taken the strategy and logic of Fabian paternalism as far as it could go, and it was found wanting. When Sidney and Beatrice Webb admired Stalin's Russia in the 1930s it was this system of providing *for* people that was so much admired. As important as the issue of efficiency in the welfare systems of bureaucratic state collectivism was the issue of the absence of rights autonomously to articulate needs and to lobby from below. Welfare recipients were objects of provision; never active subjects in defining needs and running services that met needs. The opportunity to exercise influence either through the market place or the ballot box or by direct consumer involvement was absent, except for a privileged nomenklatura layer. Kornai's concerns about the trade-off between efficiency and equality can be reformulated into a parallel statement about the trade-off between guarantees and autonomy. Here we are reminded of Jordan's (1985: 348) conclusion that:

> In future societies . . . the debate might be about . . . state services as less the expression of society's compassion and concern, or fear, of the deprived and unfortunate and more the expression of democratic participation itself – the active and politically aware involvement of equal autonomous citizens in the process of designing their societies.

We shall now turn to the problems bequeathed to new social policy makers by this legacy and outline the main policy issues to be faced in the period of transition from communism.

SOCIAL POLICY IN TRANSITION: THE ISSUES

Numerous accounts exist elsewhere (Ash, 1990; Dahrendorf, 1990; Glenny, 1990; Sword, 1990) of how the political era of bureaucratic state collectivism in Eastern Europe came to an end. Similarly there has been much discussion already of the economic problems faced by the new governments of the former Soviet Union. Here we are concerned not directly with the political and economic issues. The focus for us is the problems faced by social policy makers and those who seek to influence social policy in the period of transition. The nature of the emerging political systems and the problems associated with the marketisation of the economies will however shape both social policy and our discussion of it.

At the outset let it be said that the transition we are witnessing now in Eastern Europe and eventually in the onetime Soviet Union is the transition from what may be termed bureaucratic state collectivism to capitalism. How quickly this process will take place is not yet clear. Little state property has yet been privatised. The emerging capitalist class of entrepreneurs has yet to establish itself. Whether the transformation will be accompanied by the flowering of pluralist political democracy familiar in Western Europe also is not yet firmly established. Other non-democratic capitalist options exist. These are points addressed below and also in the section of the chapter focusing on different capitalist welfare state regime types.

The problems faced by social policy makers in the period of transition are fourfold. Each of these separate problems compounds the other, leading to an initially very bleak prospect for the establishment of a set of policies that could engender consensual support and begin to tackle and affect urgent issues.

The first problem is that the past promises of decent housing, good health services, security in conditions of sickness and old age, and other provision might now be expected to be realised and met. The old inefficient command economies could not deliver; the new market ones will be expected to. Popular expectation, combined with a heavy degree of reliance by some beneficiaries of state collectivist welfare on these services and subsidies, constitutes the first constraint on policy. The second, and related, problem is the legacy of inadequacies and inefficiencies of the past. The populations of Eastern Europe and the Soviet Union are, in general, inadequately housed, suffer more morbidity and die earlier than they need, and are often ill educated, and many live in poverty. To bring standards up to West European levels would require social policy to be given a high priority. Thirdly, and compounding cruelly the legacy of problems from the past, are the new welfare problems flowing directly from the first steps being taken across Eastern Europe towards market and eventually capitalist societies. Unemployment is already affecting 10 per cent of the workforce, except in former East Germany where the rate is much higher. The collapse of the Soviet economy, upon which Eastern Europe depended for trade, may push these figures still higher during 1992 and 1993. A new unemployment benefit system is having to be constructed and funded to meet this new situation. As prices rise, either by the impact of market forces or by decree to reflect the real value of products, wages and benefits are failing to keep pace. It is necessary for real wages and benefits to fall to match equivalent real wages for the actual market worth of the products produced in any unit of labour time. During 1990 and 1991 a fall in living standards by around 30 per cent has been common across Eastern Europe. Compensatory measures are needed, but are not often being provided, to protect the most vulnerable groups from this impoverishment. Finally, of course, there are fewer funds available to the new governments to meet these requirements constituted of popular expectation, past neglect and new problems of marketisation. Government budgets are reduced as the productive tax base shrinks and as the requirements of international lending agencies dictate.

Within and alongside this matrix of problems for policy makers two issues deserve further attention. These are the ones of justice and citizenship.

Earlier we discussed the tension and trade-off that exist between egalitarianism and efficiency, and guarantees and autonomy. These issues face East European governments and society in the period of transition in particularly sharp ways. Let us address these in turn.

Marketisation, inequality and social justice

The revolutions of 1989 were nothing if they weren't partly motivated by the wish of significant sections of the population to join in the fruits of Western capitalist consumerism. A more or less rapid introduction of market mechanisms with a pluralisation of forms of property is an inevitable outcome of these social changes. The consequences for social policy are likely to be:

1 A shift in the pattern of social inequality from one based on bureaucratic privilege to one based on market relations. There will be a consequent widening of social inequalities, which will be acceptable only in so far as capitalist conceptions of social justice replace egalitarian ones in popular consciousness. The injustices of the old regime which were so hated will give way to the more ready acceptance of some aspects of the inequality of the new regimes. There will, however, be significant sections of the working class who will continue to be attracted by egalitarian sentiments and, therefore, by a politics of levelling aimed at the restoration of the old order or something similar.
2 An incursion of market relations directly into the welfare sphere. Degrees of privatisation in the health sector, reduction in subsidy for state housing and an increase in the role of private housing, the replacement of state social security schemes by fully funded enterprise or sectoral schemes, are likely to emerge. An issue will be whether any of the previously anonymous state property will be converted into communally owned and controlled citizens' property rather than simply privatised. This marketisation process will feed new social inequalities.

An urgent issue, therefore, for policy making in this field is the determination of what would be regarded as acceptable in terms of new inequalities. What price will the poorest be expected to pay for the general expected improvements in the standard of living of all? How far should benefit levels in periods of incapacity from work reflect new wage inequalities? What minimal degree of compensation for the removal of subsidy will be politically necessary? These and comparable other bread and butter considerations of social policy makers in the West will be played out in the new situation of Eastern Europe and the Soviet Union in the 1990s.

It would be reasonable to expect the attraction of egalitarian sentiments to be stronger in some countries than in others. Relative power balances will shape the working out of these issues in each particular situation. Wnuk-Lipinski (1992) has suggested for Poland that there are those whose interests were blocked under the previous regimes who will use the new situation to satisfy their needs; whereas those whose interests were relatively well satisfied in the past will be less positive about the new emerging capitalist conception of justice. Sections of the working class and the nomenklatura who were well adapted to the old regime may favour little change. Professional groups and flexible members of the nomenklatura will find advantages in the new order. Debates between ministers of finance favouring rapid marketisations and ministers of labour and social affairs arguing for compensatory social measures reflect the settling out of these new social group and class interests.

Citizenship, civil society and welfare

The revolutions of 1989 were nothing if not symbolic of the frustration of a citizenry which demanded to have a voice in the future of their country. The articulation of social need from below and the democratic expression of such need in the political and social sphere were a hallmark of the events of 1989. There were exceptions of course. Mass movements played a much greater part in the political changes in the GDR and Czechoslovakia than they did in Hungary. In Poland the Solidarity movement had lost much of its mass character by the time it finally found itself in power. *Perestroika* was a movement of revolution from above unwelcomed by some below.

In all these countries therefore we should expect to find a social policy of the future which engages citizens much more actively in the running and controlling of policy and provision. We would expect to see a flourishing of new social initiatives of a self-help and philanthropic kind. A pluralism of welfare agencies is likely to emerge. We should expect to see a political contestation about what and whose social needs to meet.

However it would be foolish to anticipate an unproblematic ripening of an active and self-managed civil society everywhere. This is more likely in some countries than in others. There will be a differentiation of social policy between countries reflecting the differential extent to which there was a mass character of the revolutions from below in each country. There will be a differential capacity to make use of the new possibilities of citizenship between different social groups. This will feed the emergence of the new inequalities mentioned above. One of the sadder legacies of totalitarian state socialist paternalism will precisely be the dependence of significant sections of the population on the benefits of the old regime. The state will still be looked to to provide even as it gives up this role. On the other hand, the providers of welfare – doctors, teachers and lawyers – will be able to state their terms of provision.

Countries will be distinguished one from the other as to whether all, some or none of the population are ready to become active political, economic and social citizens ready to shape their own and their groups' interests. This diversity will reflect historic and cultural factors. For the Polish situation Kolarska-Bobinska (1992) has noted the low level of self-activity, communal initiative and entrepreneurial activity in the early months of 1990. Passivity, apathy, mutual dislike and hostility characterise the new situation. Wnuk-Lipinski (1992: 188) has commented:

> More freedom means greater individual responsibility for one's own life and more individualised choices of one's life career. For some this may be an unbearable burden. This is a potential social foundation of the 'escape from freedom' syndrome . . . which may result in some kind of populist movement under authoritarian leadership. To help the helpless seems to be, in this context, the most serious challenge to social policy in a post-communist society.'

Hungary presents a different picture. Bourgeois activity by citizens in the interstices of Kadarism has led to a dualised society in which one half is ready and able to become active subjects of a new welfare capitalism and the other half finds no solution to its problems in the new situation. Julia Szalai (1992) is inclined to suggest the choice is between some form of European welfare future and some form of Third Worldist future.

How the two related issues of social justice and citizenship are resolved over the coming years will be crucial in determining the broad nature of the new social policy regimes. The goal of socially just capitalist economies with flourishing civil societies within which the state reinforces the citizenship rights of the less powerful is by no means a guaranteed outcome. Under the umbrella of these two overarching issues are located a number of more specific social policy issues that will emerge and be addressed in the period of transition. Some of these are dealt with briefly below.

Women and liberation from work

Most upsetting from the standpoint of Western feminists is likely to be the ready embrace by significant sections of the female population of Eastern Europe of the opportunity to escape the double burden of work and motherhood by giving up paid work. Unemployment will encourage this process and the pressures will mount for the abandonment of the childcare and child grant arrangement which followed from the labour force requirements of the previously full employment economies.

Coupled with this will be the restoration of the influence of the Church and the threat this will pose to the liberal abortion policies. A countervailing pressure will, of course, be the possibility of the emergence of new autonomous women's movements across Eastern Europe; but the speculation must be that these will be slow in ripening.

Unemployment, poverty and racism

Unemployment will be created everywhere in the former Soviet Union and in Eastern Europe. Hurried, ad hoc out-of-work donations, schemes to establish new enterprises with enterprise allowances to ex-workers, and appeals to the voluntary sector to relieve the poor will be the first response of the new governments to the problems created. There is likely then to be a considerable differentiation in policy developments between those regimes committed to a social democratic or corporatist social policy strategy, where training schemes and fully funded benefit schemes will emerge, and those more wedded to the shock therapy and rigours of market discipline, where impoverishment of the few is likely to be tolerated in the interests of the majority.

Longstanding racist sentiments as between, say, Hungarians and gypsies, newly exposed racist sentiments as between, say, Hungarian and Romanian – and even newer racist sentiments resulting from the migration of workers across Eastern Europe – are certain to flourish in the context of unemployment and impoverishment. The break-up of the Soviet Union will bring with it a myriad of ethnic clashes. A real test of the social policy of the new regimes will be whether they challenge this racism and seek to ameliorate the social consequences or whether they capitulate to it.

Health, ecology and production

The need to rescue populations from unnecessarily early death and from undue morbidity could be regarded as the paramount social policy question faced by the Soviet Union and Eastern Europe. The developments both in terms of medical care provision and in terms of preventative health policy are likely to be slow in coming. Privatisation of aspects of medical care for some will bring early access to treatment but the level of public spending required to reach the bulk of the population will not be easy to find. Certain particularly health-damaging industrial plants are likely to close quickly, but people will continue to live off the polluted soil around them. The introduction of ecologically sounder production techniques in those factories that stay open will take longer to invest in. This slow development, coupled with the new health-threatening consequences of unemployment, new poverty, growing racism and stressful speeded-up work, suggests a further decade of early mortality and excessive morbidity for parts of Eastern Europe and the Soviet Union. In a recent comparative study of Bulgaria, Poland, Hungary and the USSR, Wnuk-Lipinski and Illsley (1990: 889) concluded similarly that:

> East European countries are abandoning their non-market economies and taking a radical look at their health systems. Transition to more effective and efficient services will be difficult. They have no appropriate models, they do not possess the organisational and management skills required to establish and maintain new effective institutions; and of course they have very few resources. In the future it will be possible to measure, monitor and publish, but the bad health statistics . . . cannot quickly be turned round.'

Let us turn now to some of the social policy measures taken in the immediate aftermath of the revolutions, before going on to locate emerging trends in the typology of regime types.

TRENDS IN SOCIAL POLICY SINCE 1989

There are both common features and distinct divergences in the post-1989 social policies of Eastern Europe. This pattern is likely to be the case within the reconstituted Soviet Union as well. These common and divergent features are catalogued more fully in Deacon *et al.* (1992). These common features might be summarised as:

- Adhocism in the development of services for the new unemployed and in the means of compensating employees and social security recipients for rapid inflation.
- Appeals to philanthropy and voluntary effort to fill the gaps left by the withdrawal of state services.
- The rapid removal of subsidies on many goods and services, including housing, with little anticipation of the social consequences for those unable to pay.
- The privatisation of some health and social care provision (though this does initially appear very limited).
- The development of independent social initiatives in the sphere of social care but with evident differential capacity of citizens to participate in these.
- The desecularisation of education and pluralisation of control over schools and colleges.
- The erosion of women's rights to childcare benefits and services and free legal abortions (although it is too early to tell how far this is developing).

- The deconstruction of the state social security system in favour of fully funded social insurance funds.
- The abolition of many health and recreational facilities provided by firms for their employees and/or their conversion into local community or private facilities.
- The ending of privileged access by virtue of nomenklatura status of old state-party apparatus to special clinics and services.
- An increase of local community control over local social provision but in an impoverished context.
- Tension between the limitation of social citizenship rights for certain ethnic minorities (gypsies everywhere, Turks in Bulgaria, Hungarians in Romania) on the one hand and increased autonomous articulation of ethnic minority needs on the other.
- A shift in the nature of the social inequalities in the use of and access to social provision from those based on bureaucratic/political privilege to those based on market relations.

However, some differences between countries are also evident. The concern with socialist values and the consequent juggling of justice versus efficiency, and social guarantees versus autonomy, still applies in parts of the former USSR, in Romania, Albania and Bulgaria and in parts of Yugoslavia. It does not apply to the same extent in the rest of Eastern Europe, where conceptions of justice and freedom more consistent with the development of capitalism are being articulated. The active development of a civil society and the flourishing of a democratic politics is more evident in Czechoslovakia and Hungary by comparison with Poland, where there is a greater tendency to social passivity which could feed an authoritarian populism. The Catholic Church for instance is influencing abortion policy and facilitating the growth of voluntary provision in Poland, whereas the less socially involved Orthodox Church in Bulgaria, for example, plays no such role. One may note also that the pre-war social democratic tradition in Czechoslovakia is being revitalised, a possibility denied, for example, to East Germany which was rapidly absorbed into Germany at a speed sufficient to generate economic collapse.

Let us now set these aspects of divergence into a more systematic discussion of welfare state regime types.

TYPOLOGIES OF WELFARE POLICY: WHAT'S NEW IN EASTERN EUROPE?

The social policy of the pre-1989 'communist' regimes of Eastern Europe and the Soviet Union shared distinctive characteristics (summarised in Table 9.)

which I earlier – elsewhere – described as bureaucratic state collectivist. The new social policy of Eastern Europe also has some common characteristics, despite the considerable diversity between countries. How do the characteristics of the new system compare with the different models of welfare policy that have been identified in developed capitalist societies? In particular, might there be a new model of welfare emerging out of the collapse of bureaucratic state collectivism?

There have been several attempts at classifying social policy or welfare state regime types among the developed capitalist nations. The most recent has been Esping-Andersen's (1990) threefold typology into 'liberal' welfare states, 'conservative corporatist' welfare states, and 'social democratic' regime types.

For Esping-Andersen, the questions asked and the criteria used to distinguish welfare state regime types fell into three clusters:

1 The degree of *decommodification* of provision. He asked to what extent services and benefits were available to citizens without price and not dependent on test of need, insurance contribution or work record.
2 The *distributional* impact of services and benefits. He asked to what extent the net effect of tax and benefit systems contributed to the generation of inequalities, the maintenance of existing social stratification, or the redistribution in an egalitarian direction of goods and services.
3 The *state/market* mix in pension provision. He asked to what extent pension entitlements were dependent on state systems, occupational systems or market systems.

At this stage in the unfolding of the new Eastern Europe and the Soviet Union it is clearly not possible to collect the array of data that would be necessary to replicate Esping-Andersen's study in relation to these countries. At this stage, and on the basis of the accounts of the development of policy described earlier, we can only begin to suggest whether the countries of Eastern Europe and the Soviet Union are likely to fall into one of his three regime types or whether a new post-bureaucratic state collectivist regime type might be emerging.

The *old system* was highly decommodified, although benefits were dependent on work record. This had a particular and unique impact on distribution in that it combined explicit and open redistributive and egalitarian practices characteristic of social democratic regime types with implicit and hidden corporatist conservative arrangements to protect the privileged position of the party state apparatus. The pension system was a state system, but a state system with built-in social differentiation in terms of entitlement.

The *new system*, ignoring for the moment the divergences, is being shaped precisely by its reaction to the perceived failures of the old system. Thus, in very general terms, we can say that the new system is and will become highly commodified, will generate a new system of inequalities, and will place far greater reliance on the market place for pension provision. The first and last features are already evident and require less discussion. On these two counts liberal welfare state regime type characteristics are emerging. The market and, perhaps to a lesser extent, private property have been seen by all social groups as the requirements for economic development. The state has been experienced as an oppressive totalitarian imposition. The chances for the retention of the state even in the sphere of welfare provision are not good. The alternative conceptualisation of a public responsibility for the welfare of the poor has been overshadowed by the need for everyone to learn how to thrive on their own initiative. So far, the emerging disquiet of the working class with some of the all-too-evident negative consequences of marketisation and privatisation have yet to find articulation in a new strategy for welfare that is neither the return to 'communist' statism nor the embrace of 'liberal market capitalism'. Formulations like 'workers' capitalism' and 'market socialism' have yet to translate themselves into political strategies and programmes.

The second feature requires more extensive discussion. There is an evident political and social tension between, on the one hand, liberating and generating new social inequalities which are increasingly perceived – despite the continued legacy and attractiveness for some of egalitarian sentiments – as being necessary for efficient economic development and, on the other hand, maintaining the privileged position of the threatened nomenklatura and sections of the working class. The matter is further complicated by the existence of a third system of inequality based upon pre-communist property and land relations which may be restored. Different ideologies of justice applied to all three systems of inequality. To the extent that the nomenklatura are able successfully to convert themselves into capitalist owners and entrepreneurs – and there is plenty of evidence that this is happening – then their interests and perhaps some of the interests of the old capitalist class may be served by liberal capitalist welfare policy. This is the path being followed in Hungary. However, to the extent that this is difficult or not desired by them, we may be witnessing in some countries the emergence of a modified form of conservative corporatism in which a deal is struck between some elements of the old nomenklatura and some elements of the working class to modify the free play of market forces, at the price of less economic growth, in order to secure a greater degree of state protection for both nomenklatura and skilled worker. This strategy will be heavily concealed by appeals to nationalist sentiment. Bulgaria and Romania may be taking this path, followed by parts of the former USSR and Yugoslavia. Certainly in the case of the former USSR as was there is no dispossessed bourgeois class ready to re-establish its position. The southern and Central Asian republics are most likely to conserve some of the centralised features of the past. Poland represents a potentially unique scenario in which the interests of a nomenklatura turned capitalist and a strong working class resistant to accepting some of the consequences of capitalism seem set on a course that is only resolvable through some form of authoritarian capitalism. Only in Czechoslovakia might we see the conversion of the statist legacy into a social democratic welfare policy strategy, but even here only after an initial flirtation with liberal welfare capitalism. At this stage, those arguing that social democratic welfare traditions are rooted in Czech history are dismissed as proto-communists. Meanwhile the future for the social policy of the GDR is of course bound up with the conservative corporatism of Germany.

It is a risky business but I hazard the following projection (see Table 9.3 below) for the prospects for welfare policy in Eastern Europe and the former Soviet Union in terms of a modified Esping-Andersen typology.

I suggest that, although it is still early days, a pattern of divergence in the politics of social policy is taking place. I predict that in a few years time we will be able to look back and characterise the social policy of these countries in terms that reflect Esping-Andersen's threefold typology, together with a new term that will have to be coined to describe the unique post-communist conservative corporatism of parts of the one-time USSR, Romania, Bulgaria and parts of one-time Yugoslavia. Poland remains problematic.

Using bivariant and multivariant regression analysis, Esping-Andersen (1990) has demonstrated the power of several variables to explain the divergence between his 'liberal', 'conservative corporatist' and 'social democratic' regime types. The variables he tested were as follows (means of operationalisation in parentheses):

demographic need (per cent of population over 65)
economic development (GDP)
economic growth (per cent real growth 1960–80)
working class mobilisation (left political party representation in terms of weighted cabinet share of seats, WCS)
influence of Catholic teaching on social policy (proportion of parliamentary seats)
historical impact of absolutism and authoritarianism (three-fold classification and year of universal suffrage).

Neither population structure nor GDP nor rate of growth of GDP were particularly significant in explaining the variation between developed welfare state regime types. Their explanatory power had been exhausted in the first generation of cross-national studies that had compared under-developed, middle-income and developed countries (Wilensky, 1975). Even so, there was some evidence to suggest that GDP was linked positively to liberal welfare state regime types.

Conservative corporatist regime types were more likely to exist where there was a combined and additive influence of Catholicism and absolutism. Liberal welfare regime types were more likely to exist where left political party representation was low and where, combined with this, economic growth was high. Social democratic regime types were likely to exist only where left party political power was high and Catholicism low (Esping-Andersen, 1990: 133–8).

Any initial attempt to 'test' the capacity of these variables, and others, to explain the emerging divergence between welfare state regime types in Eastern Europe and the Soviet Union is bound to be very tentative. Even a retrospective actual analysis in a few years' time will be provisional. One of the immediate problems to be faced is how the variables might be interpreted and hence measured in these very different circumstances. GDP, rate of growth and population structure present fewer problems. We might expect GDP to play a greater part in explaining variation because of the relative underdevelopment of some of the countries of Eastern Europe and the Soviet Union. A more complicated question is what is meant in the circumstances of the new Eastern Europe by 'left' political party representation in cabinet, 'Catholic party' representation in the legislature and the strength of absolutist and authoritarian tradition and practice? In terms of left political party representation, do the transformed Communist parties count along with both old and newly created social democratic parties as the only agencies of the 'left'? What about other forms of working-class strength via direct links with the nomenklatura unmediated by political party? Do the radical free democrats of Hungary, who have few links to the old trade union movement but progressive social policy ideas, count here? Where do Civic Forum and Solidarity, which have eschewed party political ideology and form but are now breaking up into parties, fit into this picture? The degree of working-class mobilisation associated with the two movements was quite different. Similar problems arise in terms of counting the number of Catholic seats where Catholicism is expressed indirectly through Solidarity in the eyes and practices of some members of the Sejm. And where does the Orthodox Church of the Balkans fit here? It is concerned less with social issues and more with scripture – and hence should not have the impact of Catholicism. Again, absolutism and authoritarian tradition present a fascinating question. Do we count the overthrow of the Czar as the end of absolutism, or has absolutist rule continued until today? Similarly in Poland there is a thread of continuity through the pre-war dictatorships and the post-war Stalinists, whereas Czechoslovakia had a longer lesson in democracy.

In addition to the problems of interpreting and measuring these variables in these new circumstances, there is the intuitive feeling that other factors which did not apply in Esping-Andersen's model are likely to play a part in shaping the social policy futures of Eastern Europe and the former Soviet Union. I would suggest that the nature and character of the 1989 revolutions is one of these. Another is the direct and indirect political impact of transnational agencies (IMF, European Community, World Bank) and the experience gained through societal learning from other countries. The new political actors of Eastern Europe are choosing between and being influenced by advisers from already existing welfare state regime types.

Table 9.3 suggests measures of the Esping-Andersen variables together with the additional character of the revolutionary process (CRP) and transnational impact (TI) as additional variables and begins to speculate on the likely emergence of welfare state regime types in each country in the light of the suggested impact of these variables. The character of the revolutionary process is self-explanatory as a variable. The transnational impact is likely to be higher where Western indebtedness is greater. For the immediate future the direction of transnational influence will be towards IMF-inspired liberal welfare policy. There is, however, the countervailing pressure that will be exerted by the wish to join the European Community, with the latter's social policy requirements.

Table 9.3, then, is an attempt to describe, predict and account for the broad sweep of social policy developments in these countries. Hungary and Yugoslavia (or at least Slovenia and Croatia) will – in the absence of highly influential labour parties, under the influence of foreign debts and with less Church involvement – gradually develop into liberal welfare state regime types. Czechoslovakia – at least the separate Czech republic – because of the mass character of its velvet revolution, and because of the longer training in democracy, is most likely to emerge eventually as a social democratic regime type. East Germany was already suited to join West Germany in a conservative corporatist regime. However, in the case of Bulgaria, Romania, the former USSR (or at least parts of it) and Serbia the prediction is for something new. Here the old language of socialism and egalitarianism is not dead, here the tradition of democracy is weak, here the extent to which the state is still looked to for strong support of worker interests is high, here the direct pull of Western consumer capitalism is less evident. A new but, historically speaking, probably temporary form of conservative corporatism may emerge. The expression 'post-communist conservative corporatism' captures the ideological and practical commitment to socialist values, the

Table 9.3 Projected welfare state regime types

Some Relevant Factors	Bulgaria	Czecho-slovakia	Germany	Poland	Hungary	Romania	Yugoslavia		USSR
							Slovenia	Serbia	
Economic development (relative scale)	Medium	High	High	Medium	Medium	Low	High	Low	Low
Working class mobilisation	High	High	Medium	High	Low	High	Low	Medium	Medium
Influence of catholic teaching on policy	None	Little	Little	High	Little	Little	Medium	None	Varied
Absolutist and authoritarian legacy	High	Low	Medium	High	Medium	High	Medium	High	High
Character of revolutionary process	Mass	Mass	Mass	Mass	Quietude	Mass	Quietude	Mass	Mass
Transnational impact (larger if indebted to West)	Medium	Medium	High	High	High	Low	Medium	Low	Medium
Welfare state regime type in 1995	Post-communist conservative corporatism	Social democratic[a]	Conservative corporatism	Post-communist conservative corporatism	Liberal capitalist	Post-communist conservative corporatism	Liberal capitalist	Post-communist conservative corporatism	Post-communist conservative corporatism

[a] The prognosis for the now separate Czech and Slovak republics is that social democratic possibilities continue to exist for the Czech republic but with Post-communist conservative corporatism more likely for Slovakia. The relevant factors for Slovakia are medium, high, medium, medium, mass medium respectively.

maintenance in power of some of the old guard, and the social deal struck with major labour interests. For Poland the situation is less clear. There seems no way that the high degree of working-class mobilisation and the level of their representation in government can combine with the high level of indebtedness, the strong influence of the Church and the weak tradition of democracy without a major conflict of class interest arising. Some form of authoritarian regime may prove to be necessary to secure the emergence of capitalism in that country.

REFERENCES

Arato, A. and Feher, F. (1989) *Gorbachev: The Debate*, London: Polity Press.
Ash, T. G. (1990) *We the People*, Harmondsworth, Middx: Penguin.
Dahrendorf, R. (1990) *Reflections on the Revolution in Europe*, London: Chatto & Windus.
Deacon, B. and Szalai, J. (1990) *Social Policy in the New Eastern Europe*, Aldershot: Avebury.
Deacon, B., *et al.* (1992) *The New Eastern Europe: Social Policy Past, Present and Future*, London, Newbury Park, New Delhi: Sage.
Esping-Andersen, G. (1990) *The Three Worlds of Welfare Capitalism*, Oxford: Polity Press.
Glenny, M. (1990) *The Re-birth of History*, Harmondsworth, Middx: Penguin.
Gorbachev, M. (1987) *Perestroika*, London: Fontana.
Jordan, B. (1985) *The State: Authority and Autonomy*, Oxford: Basil Blackwell.
Kolarska-Bobinska, L. (1992) 'Civil society and social anomy in Poland' in B. Deacon (ed.) *Social Policy, Social Justice and Citizenship in Eastern Europe*, Aldershot: Gower.
Kornai, J. (1986) *Contradictions and Dilemmas*, London: MIT Press.
McAuley, A. (1991) 'The Central Asian economy in comparative perspective', *World Congress of Soviet and East European Studies*, Harrogate, England, 21–26 July 1990.
Mezentseva, E. and Rimachevskaya, N. (1990) 'The Soviet country profile: Health of the USSR population in the 70's and 80's', *Social Science and Medicine* 31 (8) 867–77.
Sword, K. (ed.) (1990) *The Times Guide To Eastern Europe*, London: Times Books.
Szalai, J. (1992) 'Social participation in Hungary in context of restructuring and liberalisation' in B. Deacon (ed.) *Social Policy, Social Justice and Citizenship in Eastern Europe*, Aldershot: Gower.
Wilensky, H. (1975) *The welfare state and Equality*, Berkeley: University of California Press.
Wnuk-Lipinski, E. (1992) 'Freedom and equality: an old dilemma in a new context' in B. Deacon (ed.) *Social Policy, Social Justice and Citizenship in Eastern Europe*, Aldershot: Gower.
Wnuk-Lipinski, E. and Illsley, R. (1990) 'International comparative analysis: main findings and conclusions', *Social Science and Medicine* 31 (8).
Zaslavskaya, T. (1990) *The Second Socialist Revolution*, London: I.B. Tauris.

10 The Pacific challenge

Confucian welfare states

Catherine Jones

INTRODUCTION

So far, this has been a collection focused on Europe. Naturally there has been occasional – sometimes extensive – reference to North America by way of comparison, since Europeans, the British especially, are long accustomed to comparing themselves and their activities with 'counterparts' across the Atlantic. However, the fact that there has also been passing reference to Japan (Gould, and Rose in following chapter) is in a sense more significant. The intrusion, as it were, of *Japan* into European social policy discourse is still quite a novelty.

It is not difficult to see *why* Japan should be intruding. The acknowledged bottom line for all welfare states is, at last, economic performance. Hence the interest, belated one might say, grudging almost, in how the Japanese run their affairs. As yet, however, this interest does not run very deep – and scarcely extends at all to the still disreputable likes of Hong Kong, Singapore, South Korea and Taiwan. The Far East (revealing term) remains a long way off.

So far, European perceptions of this Far East and its miracle economies continue mostly negative. By Western standards – welfare state standards – the 'brash' new high performers are seen as falling short: as minimalist on welfare, maximalist on profit; the unacceptable face of capitalism indeed; unfair competition.

Japan has been shaking off this image somewhat, not least to the extent that Japanese levels of social spending – especially social security spending – have been creeping up lately in the international charts. Yet even the newfound respect for Japan remains couched in mostly negative terms. Japan commands serious attention as an economic success story because, for all the prosperity, its government still spends proportionately too much less on welfare to be accounted a Western-style welfare state.

Meanwhile the others, the so-called *little* tigers of Asia Pacific, seemingly still have a long, long haul to respectability in front of them. To date, their social spending figures – even those of 'socialist' Singapore – are not even included in the principal charts.

This may be an understandable, even predictable, set of Western reactions to 'upstart' Eastern competition. But that doesn't make the position any the less parochial, patronising and potentially costly to sustain.

This paper offers an alternative preliminary perspective on the region. Japan is the dominant force, the tiger so called. But there are also the little tigers to be considered. There may not be much love lost between these rivals, but they have more points in common than the mere fact of economic success. Indeed, it will be the contention of this paper that, together, they make up an 'own brand' of welfare states.

First, however, it is necessary to look behind the economic miracles themselves.

TIGER QUALITIES

There are *some* negatives in common. These are all places conspicuously short of natural advantage, whether in the shape of raw materials, mineral resources or even useable (as against precipitous) land. True, they all enjoy ready access to the sea and hence to maritime trading routes; but the sea can spell vulnerability as well as opportunity. Then again, they all have plenty of people – *the* basic resource – but plenty of people (especially unskilled, impoverished people) can spell liability as well as asset.

Moreover these are all people with a strong sense of insecurity – of being at the mercy of events and developments elsewhere over which they can have no control. One might think this an unlikely characteristic to ascribe to the inhabitants of modern Japan, as compared with, say, the likes of Singapore or especially Hong Kong. Nevertheless it is a quality the Japanese are most aware of in themselves. The future is not to be trusted. Who knows what it might bring and for whom? In short, these are 'here and now' societies. Time is not presumed to be on their side.

It's a far cry from the historiography of Western welfare states. Yet it is from such negatives that the 'positives' begin.

Determination

Desperation makes for motivation, both personal and collective. One could almost say the tigers took off because they had no choice, no *acceptable* choice. There was nothing to lose by going all out for economic advance – or, rather, far too much to lose by not doing so. The only way out of destitution or impending destitution – for families and societies alike – was up.

In the case of Japan, it was actually second time round industrialisation. The first economic revolution dating from the later nineteenth century had been accompanied by military expansionism – not unlike the experience of Germany. The second time round, in the wake of World War II defeat and devastation, economic redevelopment functioned as a permitted *substitute* for militarism – not least because it meant a saving on Allied (US) funds. Again there is the parallel with Germany.

The little tigers also started from a base of wartime and post-war ruin. As it happens they had all been victims of Japanese occupation: for a few devastating wartime years in the case of Hong Kong and Singapore; for much longer under Japanese overlordship in the case of Taiwan (from 1895) and Korea (from 1910). Like Japan itself after World War II, they all of them had seemingly nowhere to go but up, if they were not to *give* up.

The first of the little ones to take off in the 1950s was Hong Kong. There was desperation in abundance here. Hong Kong in the wake of China's communist revolution, host to massive influxes of refugees from the mainland, was faced with a blockade on trade with China (courtesy of the Korean War) and thus with ruin, as an over-populated entrepôt with nowhere for the bulk of its trade to go. Hence the temptation, looking back, to say that Hong Kong of all places industrialised and switched to producing its own goods for export simply because it was left with no other choice – other than mass destitution.

Not that the transformation of the Hong Kong economy within the space of a decade from the mid-1950s was altogether from scratch. There had been some industrial development before the war; there was the influx of Shanghai capital, plant and know-how (in respect of textiles especially) immediately before and after 1949. All the same, it would be hard to exaggerate the wonder of this high-speed, highly particular industrial revolution.

The emphasis was on small enterprises with low capital requirements and maximum flexibility. Cheap labour was the only significant resource; the family firm the principal means for its utilisation and motivation. Whatever the harsh realities of life in industrialising Hong Kong, there seems to have been no shortage of aspiration, *family* aspiration. By the time of the 'Cultural Revolution' riots of 1967, the Hong Kong economy had already been transformed. The world's first (and last?) industrial colony was in business – living proof that it could be done.

Meanwhile, Hong Kong's longstanding rival Singapore had been thrust into independence (1965) from its natural hinterland of Malaysia. There was heart-searching doubt as to whether this former colony could possibly survive and make a go of things alone. Once again therefore (in the language of hindsight and of Singaporean tradition), it was a case of needs-must, 'kick-start' industrialisation. Developing a manufacturing base, creating and sustaining an export drive, maximising incentives for foreign investment: such was to be the stuff of 'Singapore enterprises' under Lee Kuan Yew.

At least Singapore, like Hong Kong, had powerful commercial connections and experience to draw on. South Korea and Taiwan were much less prepared in this respect *and* starting from a lower economic base. In the case of South Korea, there was the sustained, reiterated devastation, disruption and division of war to contend with, and it took a military coup (1961) to galvanise what was left of this economy. Whereas in the case of Taiwan after the immediate trauma of relocation/re-occupation (the latter so far as native Taiwanese were concerned) there seems to have been less of an immediate, make-or-break sense of crisis.

Taiwan was not altogether new to industrialisation. Nor was the US-backed Taiwanese economy in serious immediate danger of collapse under the weight of the Nationalist presence. Eventually rather, this was a case of second-generation Chinese Nationalism in Taiwan coming to terms, from the 1960s, with the reality that the island was going to have to go it alone, politically and economically, for the foreseeable future. Hence, here too in the end, the call for all-out export-led growth.

In short, the economic miracles made sound sense in every case. It is not difficult to see why they were embarked on (if miracles can be 'embarked on' this side of the divine). The interest lies in trying to account for their success, as apparent so far. The Asian Pacific is hardly the only region of the world populated by desperate destitute people – and not every corner of even this region seems, as yet, to have mastered the 'trick of trade'. So how and why did the tigers bring it off?

Two contributory qualities stand out; one of them popular as it were, the other political.

Discipline

Japan has long struck outsiders, not to mention the Japanese themselves, as being one of the most well-behaved (certainly least crime-ridden) societies in the world. Singapore – certainly in the eyes of Hong Kong people – is marvelled at for being such a tidy, well-run place. Hong Kong may seem a jungle by comparison (not least in the eyes of Hong Kong people again), but even in tight-packed, crime-ridden Hong Kong one has to look hard, nowadays, to find the levels of (for instance) housing estate dereliction and graffiti characteristic of, say, run-down neighbourhoods in Britain. Ordinary people, once convincingly instructed or inducted, seem possessed of a propensity to behave, comply, conform, cooperate – in public at least.

These societies are all either Chinese (Taiwan, notwithstanding the distinction between mainlanders and native islanders), predominantly Chinese (Singapore and especially Hong Kong) or Chinese-acculturated from way back (Korea and Japan). Hence, amongst other attributes, they all rate as Confucian societies: Japan and Korea by affirmation; the Chinese others by sheer assumption.

The reference is of course to popular Confucianism – sets of common precepts, values, prohibitions – not to the teachings of the great philosopher and generations of his disciples in all their subtlety and refinement. Popular Confucianism, moreover, can vary somewhat in its practicalities from one place to the next. In Japan, for instance, the grand corporation has aggregated much of the significance and functions of the traditional family as originally envisaged by Confucius himself, whereas in Hong Kong it is rather the structure and composition of the all-important family which can nowadays be subject to manipulation in the interests of business.[1] Nevertheless 'Confucianism' still connotes a common set of presumptions and predispositions, not just in name.

It is the group not the individual that matters. The groups in question – families, corporations, entire societies – are structured hierarchically. They rest in principle on ascending orders of duty and obligation, and descending orders of responsibility and care. There is (or should be) a place for everyone; everyone should know his or her place and behave accordingly. It is only in the unique combination of his/her relationships to others that the individual properly exists.

So individuals are deemed to be possessed of roles and duties, never 'rights regardless'. Entitlements are a function of performance and position within the group. Seniority brings its just rewards with advancement up the hierarchy. Thus the individual's position is forever evolving, not static. Individuals 'pass through': they are impermanent, replaceable and eventually replaced. It is only the group itself which can persist.

To be sure, real life may not much approximate, nowadays, to the traditional, unchanging, deferential ideal. How could it indeed? 'Loss of ancestors' (a notable problem for Hong Kongers cut off from family graves on the mainland), female emancipation (or at any rate working wives, mothers and daughters), tight-packed accommodation, mass education, technological change, even increased life expectancy: altogether the times have not been kind to the elderly of late. Too many of them have been missing out on their just deserts.

Nevertheless the *ideal* persists. It is in the image of the well-run family or household – or indeed business – that the good society itself should be run. Hierarchy, duty, compliance, consensus, order, harmony, stability – and staying power: such are the hallmarks to be expected of good governance. Families and businesses might have their ups and downs but the management of society as a whole calls for an especial steadiness and steadfastness, for everyone's sake.

Corporationism is one word for this. Japan, Singapore, South Korea, Taiwan, even so-called minimum government, laissez-faire, colonial Hong Kong: each and every one of these has been conducted from 'take off' more or less in the manner of a grand national corporation. Corporationism not corporatism, note. There was never much evidence or likelihood of a voice for labour being inserted alongside that of government-and-establishment. It was Confucianism being adapted after all, not Confucianism overturned.

Hence the second, so-called political characteristic.

Direction

The tigers have (or have had) their qualities of governance in common irrespective of motley constitutional characteristics. Whatever the regime title, whatever the legal structures, whatever the voting arrangements if any, whatever citizen rights might be formally laid down, all have in practice functioned as exercises in 'top down consensus' by persuasion and/or imposition.

In short, Western-style politics and politicking has not come easily or fitted in easily, to the extent it has materialised at all. Public argument, rival parties propounding disparate points of view 'as of right', constructive conflict, 'legitimate disagreement', pluralistic bargaining and compromise: what could be more remote from the Confucian ideal – or more distasteful to Confucianist (*sic*) authorities in post? Open disagreement is a sign of failure of government.

To be sure, there has been mounting evidence of such 'failure' in recent years. Hong Kong young professionals, desperate for a voice in time for 1997, no longer leave it to a handful of Western expatriates to argue openly and virulently with officialdom (Jones, 1990a) Without Lee Kuan Yew at the helm (though for how long?), the Singapore People's Action Party (PAP) managed to lose an unprecedented 4 seats (out of 81) in the 1991 elections. South Koreans have meanwhile been witnessing a shift away from blatant authoritarianism to multi-party politics no less; though it is only the people of 'liberalised' Taiwan who can so far tune in to televised fisticuffs while their parliament is in session [*Economist*, 1991].

Yet few regard these latter antics as a sign of political strength, let alone stability. If the little tigers are coming of age politically, this may rather be in the sense that there are now fresh interests pressing for 'appropriate' accommodation in the hierarchy. Certainly, if the experience of Japan and the Japanese Liberal Party is anything to go by, the trappings of party political democracy do not (whatever the *intra*-party infighting) have to spell party political uncertainty at the top.

The ideal of good government remains: government with least appearance of politics; government which *absorbs* politics (King, 1975). It is the business of government to incorporate relevant interests and important strands of opinion – or else if necessary to neutralise them. Bureaucrats and their advisers thus matter in a way mere professional politicians do not.

Certainly it is as collections of officials – bureaucrats with something to offer or withhold – that governments have been perceived by ordinary people. Chinese tradition has had no place for 'government' in the abstract, certainly not for government as being somehow the property of the people. Government *is* people – ranks of officials, notables and 'community leaders' – whose reputations hinge on what it is by way of influence, patronage or threat they are perceived to possess.

So there are no axiomatic expectations of government, of what it should or should not do, of what should or should not be regarded as its proper responsibility. Government is what the members and functionaries of a particular administration make it. Yet by the same token there is nothing *in principle* that government officials might not be held responsible for, should circumstances turn sour. All-out riot has always been the rice bowl classes' ultimate resort.

Meanwhile, members of a governing administration each occupy their own positions in the national hierarchy. With the qualified exception of Hong Kong (whose governorship has long been presumed to rank *after* such as the Hong Kong Jockey Club and the Hong Kong and Shanghai Bank in order of influence), head of government amounts to head of hierarchy. Head of hierarchy means being in charge of the national household – and the national housekeeping (Jones, 1990b).

Looked at from one angle this may seem a recipe for unlimited authoritarianism. Looked at from another, it may seem a recipe for unlimited responsibility with all hell to pay, in terms of social breakdown and civil disorder, should things go wrong. In practice, it seems a recipe for pragmatic interventionism in the interests (*sic*) of economic advance.

In short: there has not been much 'undeserved' or indeed uncontrived about these economic miracles. Intrinsic to this contrivance, furthermore, has been social policy.

CONFUCIAN WELFARE STATES

'Lessons from abroad'

Confucianism never distinguished between the delivery or assurance of 'social welfare' and any other attributes of the functioning good society. Taking care of vulnerable members in accordance with need and desert was

intrinsic to proper family and community conduct. There was thus no call for
– and no concept of – free-standing specialised social welfare services, let
alone professionalised social work.

It was an approach to 'total welfare' predicated on social stability and
continuity. So it was by definition ill-equipped to cope with the upheavals
consequent on migration, industrialisation and urbanisation such as
characterised the Tigers in take-off. In this respect, Confucianism did not
travel well. Post-war Hong Kong and Singapore, *par excellence*, were
reckoned pathological *non*-societies composed of uncaring strangers –
precisely because the vast majority of inhabitants in each case were strangers
to nearly everyone they met.

Modern social services materialised as a by-product of Westernisation:
mainly American influence in the case of Japan, Taiwan and South Korea;
originally mainly British (colonial and missionary) in the case of Hong Kong
and Singapore. It is not hard to see from whence and how the inspiration
came.

It came initially by imposition – explicitly so in the case of British
colonial authority (to the extent that this concerned itself at all with matters
of 'social' import[2]); implicitly at the hands of missionaries 'travelling on the
coat tails of empire' and beyond (though certainly not to Japan[3]); implicitly
also via the sort of 'confrontational Americanisation' experienced by Japan
for instance after 1850[4] and again after 1945. But the development of ideas
and institutions did not stop still at the level of imposition.

The most accessible form of social service import was Western charity.
Nineteenth-century 'welfare adventurism' on the part of missionaries;
mid-twentieth-century international aid directed at refugees in flight from
the 'red menace' of communist China; latterday worldwide relief appeals in
aid of calamities elsewhere: what was all this but an adaptation and extension
every time of traditional Confucian values? Welfare this time for the stranger
in a strange place: there could be no objection in principle to sentiments so
worthy – merely some less worthy prejudices, perhaps, to be overcome.[5] At
the least, it was an intrusion which could provoke parallel 'defensive' local
voluntary action.[6] At the best, it could furnish useful precedents and
institutions for indigenisation thereafter.

The idea of *statutory* social provision was much harder to take, in more
senses than one. Governments were not traditionally obligated, any more
than citizens/subjects were traditionally entitled – or expectant.
Nevertheless, for pragmatists bent on securing economic transformation,
Western example could offer both models and warnings to work from.

By Western standards there was no necessary pattern to this process of
import and adaptation. There was no question of seeking to emulate a distinct
type of Western welfare state, even had such nuances been appreciated –

Table 10.1 'Tiger' social service provision as of 1989

Service	Hong Kong	Singapore	South Korea
Social security	Statutory public assistance. Special allowances (indexed) for elderly/ disabled	Discretionary public assistance. Central Provident Fund (compulsory national savings; employer (10%)/employee(25%); Medisave (hospital bills), housing deposits etc., lump sum for annuity	Discretionary public assistance. National pension (1988); insurance compulsory for individual employers/workers. Total (shared) contribution=3%; pension after 20 years
Health	Government & government-subsidised clinic & hospital services. No statutory health insurance. Extensive/expensive private medicine	Govt low-fee health service. Medisave (above) re insured + dependants in govt & private hospitals	Medical insurance-schemes for civil servants, teachers, workers, farmers. (c. 66% of pop. 1988) Govt subsidised health services (some)
Housing	47% pop. in 'government housing' (incl. home ownership). High rise.	86%+ pop. in 'government housing' (maj.=home ownership). Increasing high rise (urban))	1982 – govt house-building drives (pro urban home ownership). Increasing high rise (urban).
Education	Govt/govt-aided schools: 1033; private (us. small): 1580. Gradual expansion of free/subsidised places owing to demand. V. competitive. Curriculum/language complications.	Govt/govt-aided schools: 386; private: 4. Streaming/V. competitive. Govt-controlled curricula. Language complications. (Education = largest ministry)	Govt & private schools. 12 yrs compulsory education (7 free). Govt-controlled curricula. V. competitive; hence lottery (e.g. to high school)!
Social welfare	Social Welfare Department. Extensive subventions system. Extensive network voluntary orgs: Council of Social Service, Community Chest etc.	Ministry of Community Development (former Social Welfare Dept). Extensive network voluntary orgs: Council of Social Service, Community Chest (+ employee payroll deduction scheme).	Ministry of Health & Social Affairs. Extensive reliance on voluntary agencies + 'traditional Confucionism'. Increasing government investment.

Table 10.1 continued

Service	Taiwan	Japan
Social security	Discretionary public assistance. Labour Insurance compulsory for nearly all workers, employer (4/5), employee (1/5). Total 7%. Lump sum on retirement.	Employee social insurance (variable). 'National' back-up systems, e.g. (from 1985) universal basic pension. Employees' health insurance schemes; 'national' health insurance (e.g. via municipality) for rest.
Health	Limited compulsory worker health insurance. Separate schemes for civil servants, + teachers. 78% of econ. active (38% of pop.) Special for children/students. Limited free/subsidised services for needy. Govt + voluntary (e.g. missionary) hospitals; most hospitals=private.	Health insurances (above); mix of statutory, voluntary, cooperative & commercial facilities.
Housing	1976 – 10 yr Housing Plan, but: poor quality/ image/sites/ costly down payments. Pro home ownership. High rise (unpopular)	Govt investment in construction industry. Housing Corp. for home loans etc. Some public rental housing for needy groups.
Education	100% government schools. 9 yrs free education (+free textbooks for poor).	9 yrs compulsory education. Private *juku* (crammers) to supplement state schools. 95 national universities, 34 other 'public universities' & 331 private universities.
Social welfare	Department of Social Affairs. County welfare services. Subventions to voluntary agencies. Increasing govt investment.	Ministry of Health & Welfare. State-voluntary partnerships 'from top to bottom'. NB role of *Minsei-iin* community welfare 'volunteers'.

which for the most part was (and remains) not the case. Notwithstanding their great respect for German achievement, the Japanese did not set out to replicate the social market in Japan. Singapore's governing socialists (*sic*) never sought to emulate the output of Britain's post-war Labour government: anything but (Devan Nair, 1976). Not even (or especially) the Hong Kong civil service wished to see a British-style welfare state in Hong Kong. America's liberal 'land of opportunity' welfare state was scarcely calculated to appeal in Korea or Taiwan.

In short: Western-style social services constituted not ends but means, to be utilised and adapted as local circumstances might require.

Social policy objectives

Japan's constitution of 1947 specifies the Japanese people's right to enjoy health and a decent minimum standard of life. The Three Principles said to underlie the constitution of ROC Taiwan are Nationalism, Democracy and Social Welfare. The constitution of 'Fifth Republic' South Korea requires the state to promote 'social security and welfare' over and above guaranteeing human rights 'to the greatest possible extent'. Singapore and Hong Kong are neither of them possessed of such constitutional niceties, [7] yet have nonetheless been accumulating social policies and provisions at a conspicuous rate.

There was never any question, initially, of social investment as recompense for popular effort or desert. Nor was it a case of responding to popular demand – for there was none to speak of. The priority was rather to build or rebuild a sense of community where none – or none sufficient – was deemed to exist. 'Community' stood for order, discipline, loyalty, stability, collective self-help: all the traditional virtues deemed to be so at risk in post-war Japan – and so conspicuously lacking amongst the little tigers at their time of take-off. Without order, there could be no sustained economic growth; without economic growth there could be no future. It was in just such terms that ordinary people were to be instructed and reminded of the facts of life.

In particular, community building was about restoring the family to its role as bulwark of society and rendering the neighbourhood (e.g. the apartment block) the functional equivalent of a traditional village. They were scarcely trivial ambitions either of them and they could take some organising – often via the equivalent of unpaid official agents serving at the grass roots.

In the case of Japan for instance, the old system of *hohmen-iin* (volunteer 'area steward consultants') was replaced (1948) by an updated system of *minsei-iin* (registered volunteer 'social steward consultants') (Japanese National Committee, ICSW, 1990). In Singapore, networks of local residents' committees were established from the 1960s virtually at government dictat (Vasoo, 1986). In Hong Kong after the shock riots of 1966–7, there were high-profile, sloganised campaigns to 'Fight crime!' and 'Keep Hong Kong clean!', followed by the setting up of mutual aid committees at the level of the housing block, to act as a force for responsibility, law and order. All this in addition to a government-sponsored programme of 'family life education' (Jones, 1990a). Meanwhile, in President Park's Korea, the principles of *Saemaul Undong* ('self-help, diligence and mutual cooperation') were being preached and disseminated from a reconstructed countryside into the new constructed towns (Park, 1979). And there was 'planned change' for designated 'new communities' in Taiwan (Chao, 1988).Clearly ordinary people were too important to be left alone or taken for granted.

Nevertheless, there was another side to the picture. Ordinary people thus exposed to 'active government' could develop notions of their own importance hitherto unforeseen by either side, at the same time as government 'in the service of the economy' could increasingly be coming to mean government as a provider or sponsor of services useful to the economy. Once exposed to such services 'courtesy of government' – and to the extent they themselves perceived them to be useful – ordinary people were liable to look for more of the same; if not as a right then certainly as a perk to go for in the perennial struggle to get ahead. Just so has a popular learning exercise been taking place, beyond the bounds of any formal education programme.

So it was, in the case of the little tigers at least, that practical community building could end up as much about striking bargains as imposing grand designs. It was Sir Murray MacLehose (reforming ex-Governor of Hong Kong) who remarked in 1976, not before time, that 'people will not care for a society which does not care for them'.[8] It was Hong Kong's by then social services (*sic*) he had in mind as the basis for a *quid pro quo*: putative pillars for a new form of consensual society – not because these services (housing, education, health care) had been designed with any such end in view, but because they happened in the meantime to have proved their popularity on the ground.

To be sure, this was a defensive colonialist speaking. It would be unrealistic to expect similar frankness from government spokesmen elsewhere. Yet this scarcely signifies that the same truths do not obtain: the longer and better established the provision of popular useful services, the more people are likely to expect of them. Just so has popular housing satisfaction emerged as critical to political and social stability in Singapore (Devan Nair, 1976). Just so have business leaders in Japan been complaining in general – in true 'I told you so' fashion – that the Japanese people have grown to expect far too much of government (and of themselves as employers).

Yet it has been a learning exercise very much concerned with down-to-earth practicalities from a family point of view. Nowhere, for instance, has there been a popular call for 'social justice Western style' – let alone for actual income redistribution in the cause of say 'equality' or 'citizen's rights'.

Useful services (Table 10.1)

The most popular service, from the point of view of governments and peoples alike, has been education: scarcely a Western import in itself, however much form and content may have been influenced (positively and otherwise) by Western example. Schooling ranks as the single most important item go-ahead families are wont to invest in, with or without government help. So persuading parents to send their children to school has never been much of a problem. The problem has rather been one of reconciling parental hopes and demands with system capacity and perceived national requirements.

Respect for learning is traditional; but no less traditional is the perception of education as instrumental to family fortune.[9] The parental ideal (apparently also the employer's ideal in Japan at least) is for an academic education of the sort (and extent) to command prestige and thus open doors to a promising career. Traditionally again, prestige is only to be acquired via competition; so today's parents (and others) tend to value forms of education and educational institution according to the number and difficulty of exams required to qualify for entry. But governments may be less concerned with exams for exams' sake and more concerned with manpower needs. The scope for mismatch is obvious.

Perhaps its ultimate embodiment is, strangely enough, to be found in Japan where, once entry has been secured to a sufficiently prestigious university after years of exam-dominated schooling both in and out of school hours, [10] the happy, successful university student has allegedly nothing very serious to do during the closing years of his formal education, until the time comes to take up the well-earned safe job.[11]

Much the same sort of outlook lies behind the proliferation of government-aided Anglo-Chinese grammar schools in 'consumer-led' Hong Kong, at the expense of other forms (not least traditional Chinese forms) of secondary education. Hence the proliferation here, it is alleged, of semi-literate 'worst of all worlds' teachers and pupils whose grasp of English is minimal and whose proficiency in Chinese barely rudimentary.[12] In the case of Singapore it has prompted a less defensive government to impose (1980) a system of streaming on all schools, whereby degrees of ability are first identified by examination at the end of 'primary three' and educational schedules thence distributed accordingly. In the case of South Korea, most intriguingly, it has led to the imposition of lotteries to help determine entry to middle school, high school and now at last university – so destructive (and expensive for parents faced with the extra tutoring bills) had the examinations hell become.

By contrast, two other sorts of popular service are of anything but traditional appeal. Rather the popularity of housing and (Western-style) health care has been of governments' own making, most notably of those governments in charge of Hong Kong and Singapore. In each case the initial (colonial) concern was simply with public health and safety as a prerequisite for economic viability. Too much dirt and disease was bad for trade; urban squatters constituted a fire and riot hazard (quite apart from taking up valuable development land); orphans (not to mention 'orphaned parents') cost money to support. Just so did Hong Kong's post-war administration become convinced of the need, not merely for a basic public health/health education service, but for a mass public housing programme.

It was to prove an embarrassing success story. So popular does (cheap) Western medicine become there are soon charges of 'cultural inequity' from the proponents of traditional Chinese medicine, as the colony's medical and health department struggles to keep pace (never to catch up) with the mounting demand for its services. Then again, once the design of mass resettlement estates – never intended as an exercise in housing provision so much as an aid to squatter clearance – was even marginally improved in the interests of health and safety, they too took on the aura of a desirable (cut-price) public provision.

In both Hong Kong and Singapore it was a case of governments reacting pragmatically to pressures of population and circumstance such as threatened to overwhelm any prospects for order and (hence) prosperity. However, in the case of People's Action Party Singapore, the notion of mass public housing provision was associated from the start not just with physical development but with the notion of 'rooting' an otherwise unpredictably rootless population within the boundaries of the state. Hence the emphasis on public housing for purchase (with help from the Central Provident Fund, see below), a strategy now being pursued in Hong Kong too, in would-be defiance of 1997.

Without comparably sudden and dramatic pressures of population to contend with, the level of government involvement in housing amongst the other little tigers has been much less. Taiwan's first Ten Year Housing Plan dates only from 1976; Korea's (five-year) Socio-Economic Development Plan includes a mass *urban* housing component only from 1982. In both cases, significantly, the emphasis was again to be on housing for purchase – and in both cases first results were disappointing not least, in the case of Taiwan, because the units produced were too poor and/or too badly located to attract purchasers (Chan, 1988). In other words, the useful service (from the point of view of town planning) wasn't useful enough (from the point of view of consumers).

Meanwhile Japan continues to stand out both for the poorest quality of housing (relative to living standards and cost) and paucity of public provision in this respect. Whatever else the promise of a 'decent minimum standard of life' for every Japanese might include, housing has clearly not been a prime part of the deal; it is not something people have come to expect (or have had a chance to expect) government to guarantee.

It is for occupational social security cover that Japan stands out. Pensions, health insurance, unemployment protection, even help with home purchase: for those in mainstream employment, especially with a major corporation, quality of career very much spills over into quality of social entitlements. To be sure the 'Japanese welfare society' guarantees everyone nowadays a 'decent' basic pension, plus 'basic' health insurance (not usually extending to sick pay) via an assortment of local and national arrangements for those not otherwise protected, together with 'basic' unemployment compensation.[13] But it's still much better in every way to be in a good job for life – for all of one's working life.

It is significant that one – if not *the* – topic of social concern in contemporary Japan centres on the implications of a fast-ageing population structure for the future of the social security system. 'Had we thought sufficiently ahead, ' critics argue, 'the pension reforms of the 1970s would never have been embarked upon'.[14] As it is, the formula for determining future benefits in relation to contribution records has since been toned down (1985), yet the worry remains (Japanese National Committee, ICSW, 1990).

It is a worry that the little tigers, possessed of their own ageing populations, readily comprehend. Central to all of their calculations – not just those of futureless Hong Kong – has been the maxim that one should never bank on the future; that one should not saddle government or industry with burdens and commitments not capable of adjustment (or abandonment if need be) as circumstances may require.

In the case of Hong Kong it has meant the denial of social insurance altogether, in favour of a system of non-contributory allowances (backed up by public assistance), which in practice assures the current elderly and disabled a relatively secure standard of living by regional standards (Jones, 1990a, b). Elsewhere it has meant 'social insurance' systems geared overwhelmingly to short-term risks and (in the case of the elderly) one-off payments. Apart from Medisave to help with hospital bills, Singapore's Central Provident (i.e. compulsory employer-worker savings) Fund ensures the availability of lump sums in aid of house purchase (for instance) and to cushion retirement.[15] Likewise there is worker social insurance in Taiwan to cater for sickness and health care needs but, again, to offer only a lump sum in case of retirement. Of all the little tigers, only Korea has so far declared itself (1973, confirmed in 1988) in favour of a system of compulsory wage-related pensions insurance – and even in this novel case, the level of contributions has been pitched so low as to suggest the eventual pensions must be modest by anyone's standard.

Social security – in the fullest sense of the term – is seen as dependent in the last resort not on governments but on families and communities; on voluntary action, both formal and informal; on traditions revived and reinforced in many respects by Western example. Aside from the appetite for education, the attachment to non-statutory social welfare constitutes the most striking common Confucian welfare state characteristic.

Moreover this is a mainstream characteristic, not just a residual attribute. Voluntary action (paid and unpaid) is not left a matter of chance. It can be orchestrated, coordinated, subsidised, regulated, advised, directed, quality-controlled – to an extent Western agencies, mindful of their freedoms even as they compete for public funding and recognition, might find incomprehensible. But then the importance of the statutory-voluntary distinction *per se* remains very much a Western idea. The Japanese social welfare system for instance interwines statutory and voluntary agencies and responsibilities, paid and unpaid, literally from top to botttom (Japanese National Committee, ICSW, 1990). The Hong Kong Social Welfare Department's programme plans depend for the bulk of their operation on the work of voluntary agencies paid for out of public funds according to agreed statutory formulae (Jones, 1990a).

Not that private fund raising need be left to chance either – witness the efforts to inculcate charity-mindedness amongst the peoples of Hong Kong and Singapore via massive annual Community Chest campaigns ('The Community Chest serves our community best!') and a 'voluntary' payroll deduction scheme in aid of the Community Chest, respectively. The fund-raising results of such efforts could be dramatic, though not everyone was convinced this was genuine charitable sentiment being evoked – so much as a wish to preserve or acquire social respectability.

But then the social workers frequently responsible for voicing such home-truths could themselves be in an uncertain position. Theirs is a new profession still finding its level and very much in search, therefore, of status supports. Hence the eagerness to impress 'upwards' that they are no 'free lunch merchants' and to demonstrate 'downwards' that they are indeed capable of delivering the goods to ordinary people who turn to them for help or advice.[16] There is not much scope or call here for the likes of non-directive case-work, axiomatic championing of the underdog or mere, sheer 'enabling' community action.

CONCLUSIONS

This is welfare capitalism for sure. But whether it counts as a form of welfare statism depends on how policy specific or otherwise the attributes of welfare statism are taken to be. None of the tigers would qualify by Richard Titmuss' standard of a welfare state, for instance, since manifestly none of them are committed to his 'institutional-redistributive' model of social policy as the ultimate objective. Yet once a more variegated set of criteria in respect of a range of different types of welfare state is allowed – even insisted on – it becomes much more difficult to exclude the tigers, any of them, from this particular club.

There has been recurrent reference in the present collection to just such a typology (variously modified) of welfare states (e.g. Esping-Andersen, 1990). It is very much a *Western* welfare capitalist typology. As such, it serves well to establish what the tigers are not. They are not liberal: there is far too much social direction and too little sense of individual rights (including minimal social rights) for this label to be applied, even in vaunted 'capitalist paradise' Hong Kong. Manifestly they are not social democratic either. Nor, given the absence of sufficient status-preserving statutory social benefits to accommodate the aspirations of the employed 'middle classes' for instance, are they to be accounted conservative corporatist; though this category comes closest to the mark.

Thus, just as Deacon for instance has found it appropriate to specify additional categories in order to accommodate Eastern Europe (see above pp. 191–7), so it seems appropriate in this case to add another composite category: that of the *Confucian* welfare state. Conservative corporatism without (Western-style) worker participation; subsidiarity without the Church; solidarity without equality; laissez-faire without libertarianism: an alternative expression for all this might be 'household economy' welfare states – run in the style of a would-be traditional, Confucian, extended family (Jones, 1990b).

So much for the typecasting of tendencies to date – but what of the future? To what extent are determination, discipline and direction likely to continue as hallmarks of tiger performance? Might the attractions of wealth and/or welfarism serve to modify the mix over time? Alternatively (or conjointly) might the force of the Asian Pacific example stamp itself, as it were, on welfare state Europe?

Certainly there are danger signs apparent to anxious local observers on the first count. There has been much public criticism, for instance, of today's young adult Japanese (deprived incidentally of the responsibilities of early home ownership, thanks to rocketing house prices at any rate within the Tokyo area) as an irresponsible, pleasure-loving, leisure-seeking, altogether frivolous and disrespectful generation. Elsewhere and seemingly more seriously, Hong Kong's young 'social professionals' demand a say in policy making *in the interests* (so it is said) of ordinary people, whilst students in South Korea are still (incredibly) rioting for revolution and re-unification with the North. Nothing looks all that safe to their elders and betters, in every case.

But since when have the old been disposed to approve or trust in the young? Two points – one general, one particular – are worth bearing in mind. First the particular. Hong Kong faces its climacteric of 1997 and South Korea is currently engaged in potentially momentous negotiations with its North. It would be a strange generation of young people in either case which (permitted at least some freedom of expression) did not evince anxiety and some wish to participate in determining its own future. But this is hardly proof in itself of fundamental, permanent disaffection. Which brings us to the second, general point: young people, barring accidents, grow older; they acquire responsibilities and expectations which – other things being equal in these of all societies – should lessen or at least *transfer* the grounds for dissatisfaction from one year and one generation to the next. It is not as if Western welfare statism, as caricatured right across Asia Pacific, had ever appealed as a system (*sic*) to emulate – as against to exploit.

Meanwhile what price or chance convergence in an opposite direction? Japanese styles of management have long attracted attention and support whenever they have spelt jobs in Britain ('gateway to Europe') for instance. Appeals for a leaner, more family-and-*community*-oriented welfare state in Britain might almost have been culled from Japanese (not to mention even Hong Kong) example in any case. The European Economic Community has long been accused (not least by one-time leading lights of Britain's Labour Party[17]) of putting capitalist economics before all else. So, if greater competitiveness is what is called for, why not a variant of Confucianism for Europe?

Of which of course there is no chance – for the same reason that (even) the welfare states of Europe are currently finding it so difficult to agree amongst themselves, within and without the present EC, about what the 'social face of Europe' ought to look like and at whose say-so. Welfare states are born not made, for all the benefits and tips to be derived from greater mutual awareness and understanding of the alternatives, near and far.

NOTES

1 'Utilitarianistic familism' according to S.K. Lau (1982).
2 Even in no-nonsense nineteenth-century Hong Kong, for instance, it proved necessary to invest in public health reform if this 'haunt of fever' was ever to pay its way as a trading station.
3 Under the Tokugawa Shogunate (1600–1853) Christian missionaries – and the practice of the Christian religion – were prohibited in Japan, on pain of death.
4 It was actually in 1853 that US Commander Perry sailed his famous squadron of warships into the fortified harbour of Uraga.
5 cf. Richard Titmuss' insistence that 'giving to the anonymous other' was the ultimate test of altruism (Titmuss, 1970).

6 e.g. the famous Tung Wah Chinese Hospital (nowadays a chain of charitable establishments) was founded in Hong Kong in 1870 in part response to Western expatriate 'provocation' (Jones, 1990a).
7 Though the Basic Law for post-1997 Hong Kong does imply continuity in social welfare policy (Jones, 1990a).
8 Address at Opening Session of the Legislative Council, 6 October 1976.
9 Note the age-old Chinese tradition of entry to the Mandarinate by competitive examination.
10 Enrolment at a private *juku* after school being a virtual *sine qua non* for success.
11 'British university students take jobs in the vacations. Japanese university students tour the world in vacations and take jobs from the start of the autumn term.' Personal observation vouchsafed to author, Tokyo 1990.
12 Note that the mastery of Chinese characters (c. 6,000 for everyday newspaper readership, 20,000 for book reading, 60,000 or so for true scholarship) was not the sort of time-undertaking to be compared with learning the western alphabet!
13 e.g. lump-sum compensation for seasonal workers and those aged 65+.
14 In 1973 a new wage-related 'pension standard' was set for both the employees pension and the national pension. Henceforth the average pension in payment was to be equivalent to about 60 per cent of the average wage, and indexed to consumer prices.
15 Under the 'Minimum Sum' scheme from 1987, retirees can now be compelled to leave part of their lump sum in the Fund – or to deposit it with a bank – so as to guarantee a measure of continued income after age 55.
16 This last is a role they have been performing with some success in Hong Kong of late: witness their electoral successes in respect of District Boards and then the Legislative Council.
17 Witness the Euro-Referendum campaign of 1975.

REFERENCES

Chan, Hsiao-Hung Nancy (1988) 'Public housing development plan: experience in the Republic of China' in P.C. Lee (ed.) *Dimensions of Social Welfare Transition: Sino-Brtish Perspectives*, Taipei: Chu Liu Book Company.
Chao, W. (1988) 'Planned change in community development: its application in Taiwan' in P.C. Lee (ed.) *Dimensions of Social Welfare Transition: Sino-British Perspectives*, Taipei: Chu Liu Book Company.
Devan Nair, C.V. (1976) *Socialism That Works . . . The Singapore Way*, Singapore: Federal Publications.
Economist Magazine (1991) Supplement, 'Where tigers breed: a survey of Asia's emerging economies', 16 November.
Epsing-Andersen, G. (1990) *The Three Worlds of Welfare Capitalism*, Cambridge: Polity Press.
Japanese National Committee, International Council of Social Work (ICSW) (1990) *Social Welfare Services in Japan*, revised edn, Tokyo.
Jones, C.(1990a) *Promoting Prosperity: The Hong Kong Way of Social Policy*, Hong Kong: Chinese University Press.
—— (1990b) 'Hong Kong, Singapore, South Korea and Taiwan; oikonomic welfare states', *Government & Opposition* 25 (4), Autumn, 447–62.

King, A.Y.C. (1975) 'Administrative absorption of politics in Hong Kong', *Asian Survey* 15 (5), May, 422–39.

Park, C.H. (1979) *Korea Reborn: A Model for Development*, Englewood Cliffs, NJ: Prentice Hall.

Titmuss, R.M. (1970) *The Gift Relationship: From Human Blood to Social Policy*, London: Allen & Unwin.

Vasoo, S.(1986) 'Residents' organisations in the new towns of Hong Kong and Singapore: a study of social factors influencing neighbourhood leaders' participation', PhD thesis, University of Hong Kong.

Part IV

On the state of the argument

11 Bringing freedom back in

Rethinking priorities of the welfare state

Richard Rose

> In socialist countries the discussion of individual freedom was an ideological taboo for decades; notions such as 'individualism' or 'liberalism' had strong pejorative connotations. But I am convinced that respect for individual freedom is not only compatible with the original aims of many socialist thinkers but should become a fundamental ingredient of the social programme everywhere.
>
> (Janos Kornai, *Vision and Reality, Market and State*, 1990: 215)

Is welfare defined solely by activities of the state or can it exist independently of state action? Conventional studies of the welfare state often imply the former view. However, any study of goods and services of primary importance to the majority of individuals must consider non-state as well as state sources of welfare. The collapse of centrally planned systems of welfare in Eastern Europe[1] is a reminder of the need to think clearly about the dependence of welfare upon the state. Since East European regimes imposed by the Soviet Union were dictatorships, it is also necessary to examine the relation between freedom and state welfare, for, even if East Europeans have had a modicum of state welfare provision, they have not been able to take freedom for granted.

In the abstract, we can define total welfare in the family (TWF) as the sum of goods and services produced by the household (H), the market (M) and the state (S) (Rose, 1989: ch. 8).

$$TWF = H + M + S$$

This perspective includes, regardless of source, the goods and services essential to the majority of households, such as income, food, housing, personal social services, education, health and transportation.

Conventional studies of the rise of the welfare state posit a unilinear shift from the production of welfare in the household to production by the market, and then the fiscalisation or *étatisation* of welfare. Although the intent is not totalitarian, the thrust is clear: welfare expands with increased involvement by the state in the production and distribution of welfare.

Historically, the role of the state was to produce order, not welfare as that term is understood in contemporary social science (Rose, 1976a). Order can be produced through coercion or through democratic institutions; most member states of the United Nations today are authoritarian rather than democratic in their orientation. Welfare can also be produced by democratic or by authoritarian regimes. Democracy is neither a necessary nor a sufficient condition for the provision of education, health care and social security. Although the welfare state is *not* a road to serfdom, for four decades Soviet-style regimes from East Berlin to Siberia demonstrated that a welfare state can deny civil and political rights, and defend such actions, as Kornai notes, in terms of collectivist values.

Freedom *must* be brought in when we consider welfare in Europe today, for a political revolution is transforming state, market and society in formerly centrally planned economies that were dependent upon the power of an authoritarian regime. Social scientists must bring freedom back into their thinking, if they wish to remain scientists (that is, persons interested in ideas not restricted to a single or a few societies). Cities such as Prague, Budapest and Dresden are older than the cities of the British Industrial Revolution, and Central Europe has been central to European history much longer than the offshore island of Britain.

The object of this chapter is to examine basic relations between the state, welfare and freedom in democratic and non-democratic political systems. The first section demonstrates that it is possible to have rights without welfare, and welfare without rights. The implications of a non-democratic inheritance for post-Communist East European societies is shown in the second section. The conclusion asks: if forced to choose, what priority would we give to freedom as against material benefits from the state?

RIGHTS WITHOUT WELFARE AND WELFARE WITHOUT RIGHTS

Since the welfare state is a political as well as a social institution, it has two sets of attributes. The welfare criterion distinguishes between social benefits that are state-based or market-based. It is also necessary to distinguish between countries in which civil and political rights are granted to the great majority of citizens, and those in which they are not. Bringing freedom back in thus produces four logically possible relationships between political rights and social benefits (Figure 11.1).

Within states that grant democratic political rights, there is a clear contrast between Scandinavian countries that provide a very high standard of social

Political rights

| | Yes | No |

Social benefits

	Yes	No
State-based	Democratic welfare state (e.g. Britain)	Undemocratic welfare state (USSR)
Market-based	Democratic states with welfare in society (e.g. Japan)	Undemocratic states with welfare in society (Asian NICs)

Figure 11.1 Alternative dimensions of rights and welfare

benefits, and the United States and Japan, where the role of the state is much less. Among newly industrialising third world nations, few are democratic, and the great majority expect their subjects to rely upon the market or the household for welfare. Soviet countries were exceptional in combining authoritarianism with welfare state programs, a characteristic shared with some non-democratic oil-rich sheikdoms in the Middle East.

Both rights and welfare: the British experience

The classic analysis of the relation between politics and welfare in Britain is T.H. Marshall's essay on *Citizenship and Social Class*. He defined citizenship as 'a kind of basic human equality associated with the concept of full membership of a community' (Marshall, 1950: 8f.); full membership conferred three distinctive sets of rights:

1 *civil*: the rights necessary for individual freedom – liberty of the person, freedom of speech, thought and faith, the right to own property, and to conclude valid contracts, and the right to justice.
2 *political*: the right to participate in the exercise of political power, as a member of a body invested with political authority or as an elector of the members of such a body.
3 *social*: the right to a modicum of economic welfare and security, the right to share to the full in the social heritage and to live the life of a civilised being according to the standards prevailing in the society.

Linking civil and political with social rights involved a normative as well as a positive set of concerns. Marshall was not just trying to advance a positivist hypothesis that 'politics matters'; he was also painting a picture of a society that had achieved its highest (and, implicitly, ultimate) level of civic virtue.

By contrast, American social scientists have tended to adopt a non- or anti-normative stance, concentrating upon welfare in material terms only. This was implicit in Frederick Pryor's (1968: 285) functionalist conclusion to a comparison of East and West European welfare systems: 'the policy dilemmas facing decision makers are quite similar in all nations regardless of system', and Wilensky's (1975: 48) conclusion that 'ideology consistently adds nothing' to an understanding of welfare outcomes.

Contemporary advocates of a written constitution and a bill of rights similarly incorporate social welfare benefits as fundamental in government. The elaborate draft constitution produced by the Institute for Public Policy Research (1991: Article 27) lists the right of everyone to an adequate standard of living, including adequate food, clothing, housing, social security and education. However, the IPPR document adds: 'The provisions of this Article are not enforceable in any court.' By making social rights non-justiciable, it thus recognises that social rights do not have the same status as civil and political rights (see Rose, 1976b).

Marshall's categories appear as part of a natural evolutionary process, or even as if social rights were caused by the expansion of civil and political rights. However, sequence does not prove causation. Heclo (1974: 288f.) argues that the introduction of the welfare state in Britain had more to do with the activities of elites than with enfranchisement and popular demands, and in Scandinavia middle-class interests provided much of the initial impetus for the welfare state (Baldwin, 1990). Civil and political rights are liberal, granting individuals freedom from arbitrary state action. The welfare state is a collectivist institution, mutualising costs and benefits through the state's powers of taxation and capacity to provide benefits without charge. As Swann (1988: 10f.) emphasises, the collectivising process still operates very much through external compulsion and does not rely on the self-steering capacities which human beings may possess; education continues to be imposed on children and social security taxes on works. The juxtaposition is not fortuitous.

Money is seen as the main constraint upon social rights. This is recognised in the IRPP's refusal to give courts the authority to compel an elected government to allocate revenue to maintain 'adequate' social welfare standards in the face of fiscal difficulties.

A lack of accountability of service providers is a second constraint upon social rights. It arises from the fact that state-funded social benefits are provided on a non-market basis. They are free of the personal ties involved in the provision of services in the household, and of consumer choice in the market. As Day and Klein (1987) have shown, popularly elected office-holders are unable to hold accountable the experts who actually deliver services to individuals in health, education and personal social services. The non-market provision of social services by the state gives experts or 'street-corner bureaucrats' the effective power to determine access to many social benefits through queuing, labelling or discretionary decisions (Lipsky, 1980).

Marshall adduced concepts in principle applicable to all advanced industrial nations, and sociologists elsewhere have taken up his ideas (see e.g. Lipset, 1965; Bendix and Rokkan, 1964). Yet the essay starts with Maitland's *Constitutional History of England*, and the story told is English, in Shakespeare's sense (Richard II, ii):

> This happy breed of men, this little world,
> This precious stone set in the silver sea,
> Which serves it in the office of a wall,
> Or as a moat defensive to a house,
> Against the envy of less happier lands,
> This blessed plot, this earth, this realm,
>   this England.

However, the account of the evolution of rights does not even fit the history of the United Kingdom. Civil and political rights were never as secure in Ireland as in England before 1921 or in Northern Ireland thereafter. The evolution of social welfare in Ireland since it became independent has flowed in a different direction from the stream of English history, reflecting Catholic, not liberal doctrines (see Rose and Garvin, 1983). Hence, to understand the welfare state as a general idea, we must identify alternatives to the British experience.

Rights without welfare

The struggle for civil and political rights, in Isaiah Berlin's (1969) classic sense of freedom from the authority of an oppressive state, lasted far longer in Europe than in England, and the alternatives were far harsher. Democratic regimes were institutionalised in Western Europe between the beginning of this century and 1945, in Southern Europe in the past quarter-century, and in Eastern Europe the process is only now commencing.

The European Community makes respect for civil and political rights a primary condition of membership. The European Convention on Human Rights and the European Court of Justice give individuals justiciable claims for political and civil rights. However, agreement about political and civil rights is not matched by agreement about the definition or material value of social rights. This has been made evident in the debate between proponents and opponents of incorporating provision for a 'Social Europe' within the Single European Market (see Teague, 1989; Teague and Grahl, 1991).

Table 11.1 Public expenditure on social programmes by EC member states

	As % GDP
Belgium	34.9
France	34.2
Denmark	33.9
Netherlands	30.7
Italy	26.4
Ireland	26.1
Germany	25.2
UK	20.6
Greece	19.5
Portugal	18.6
Spain	17.0

Source: OECD (1989) *OECD in Figures*, Paris: OECD pp. 16f, 22f.
Notes: No social expenditure data for Luxembourg. Portuguese figure is an estimate.

If the percentage of gross domestic product spent by government on social policy is used to measure commitment to social rights, then the highest-ranking nation, Belgium, makes more than twice the effort of the lowest-ranking nation, Spain (Table 11.1). Differences among these advanced industrial nations cannot be ascribed to lower levels of development, for Germany and Britain rank below average, and Ireland and Italy above in public spending on social policy. Differences reflect conflicting priorities of elected governments.

The European Community can make respect for priceless civil and political rights a condition of membership, but it cannot confer upon its 320 million citizens a right to equal benefits in education, health care and social security, for there is no political consensus for the massive redistribution of income that this would require between Northern and Southern Europe, and in future between Western and Eastern Europe. There is not even a consensus about what the appropriate standard of social welfare ought to be. To treat the average EC level of social expenditure as desirable would require big cuts in countries such as France and Denmark. To set the standard at the level of the biggest spender would require massive tax increases in 11 other nations.

From the United States to Australia and Japan, there is ample evidence that civil and political rights are not a sufficient condition for the state provision of high levels of social benefits (Rose, 1991a). The United States was a constitutional democracy for almost a century and a half before the federal government took the first steps toward providing social security, and half-measures for health care came later still. Japan is another example of a society that enjoys a high level of well-being, yet it ostentatiously rejects the values of the welfare state, and the Japanese rely far more upon households and markets.

Logically, there is no necessity for the state to provide social benefits for, in the language of economics, the prototypical benefits – education, health care and old age pensions – are private goods that are capable of being sold in the market, and those who do not pay for them (or have charges paid by a third party) can be excluded. Public goods such as military defence and clean air are collective goods; there is no basis for excludability, and thus of charging for defence or for clean air (see e.g. Walsh, 1987).

Economic growth is the *sine qua non* condition for increased welfare in society. A prosperous market economy is consistent with a high level of private sector *or* state provision of welfare, or with a mixture of resources in a 'mixed' society. If one thinks of maximising total welfare rather than just publicly financed welfare, then America and Sweden are similar in what is spent on health care as a percentage of GDP, 10.8 per cent in the United States and 9.6 per cent in Sweden. Britain demonstrates the truth of the old adage that if you don't have it you can't spend it, for it spends much less per person on health care than either of these wealthier societies (OECD, 1985: Tables 1, 2).

Even when GDP per capita is high, it does not follow that all the conditions are met for the effective state provision of social benefits. Three conditions are independent of fiscal resources: (1) a sense of social solidarity consistent with national citizenship; (2) trust in the benign behaviour of the state; and (3) belief in the efficacy and honesty of state action. Across nations, each condition is a variable. A disjunction between social solidarity and citizenship is evident in the United States, where race, ethnicity, religion, class and region segment the population, leaving citizenship a residual social status conferring only residual social benefits. In Mediterranean societies citizens assume that the state is inefficient, corrupt or both; there privatisation can be a 'good government' rather than a right-wing concept. In Eastern Europe repressive regimes lacking popular support have been widely distrusted by most citizens.

Welfare without rights

A German-oriented approach to the development of the welfare state is more appropriate in this context than an Anglo-centric view, for Wilhelmine Germany was first in introducing programmes now regarded as the core of the welfare state. Even the liberal progenitors of the welfare state in Britain looked to pre-democratic Germany for ideas.

The welfare state is not the consequence of democracy but, as Flora and Heidenheimer (1981: 23, 46) argue, 'a far more general phenomenon of modernisation; not exclusively tied to its "democratic-capitalist" version'. A modernising state may promote social welfare benefits as part of a strategy of 'authoritarian defence', *substituting social rights for political or civil rights*. This was the strategy of Bismarck, and even more that of the National Socialism of the Third Reich.

In the post-1945 era, East European countries have further demonstrated that it is possible to adopt welfare state policies without being a democracy. Communist regimes were formally committed to the universalistic provision of education, health care and social security through the state. The public provision of social benefits was entirely consistent with the collectivisation of the economy. Non-market allocation of private welfare benefits paralleled the non-market allocation of goods and services considered private sector activities in Western societies.

To paraphrase Margaret Thatcher's assertion, 'There is no such thing as society', East European regimes acted on the ideological assumption that there is no such thing as the individual or the family – and did so far longer and with far more force than the Thatcher administration commanded. Communist ideology denied the existence of civil society, that is, institutions providing welfare independently of the state. In consequence, reliance on non-state resources was a form of alegal or 'anti-regime' activity (see Shlapentokh, 1989). The absence of political and civil rights made it possible for these regimes to marginalise non-state sources of welfare.

In actuality, the economic deficiencies of the non-market economies of Eastern Europe created permanent shortages, thus depriving citizens of the level and variety of welfare services that developed simultaneously in Western Europe. Kornai (1990: 216ff, 235) demonstrates how the absence of individual freedom was counterproductive in instrumental as well as intrinsic terms, for the shortages of welfare services were compounded by the power given to non-accountable bureaucrats to ration scarce welfare services. In default of market alternatives, the result was:

> a somewhat perverse combination of bureaucratic rationing and veiled commercialisation. The mere fact that medical care is free of charge to every citizen does not make patients satisfied, since the quality of service is frequently substandard. Besides there is substantial disaffection amongst the doctors and the medical staff. The widespread occurrence of 'gratitude money' is a peculiar signal of many people's willingness to spend more of their own money on their health directly.

Neither welfare nor rights

Most member states of the United Nations neither guarantee civil and political rights nor provide social benefits. This is true of New

Commonwealth countries with a Westminster heritage, as well as of states with other origins.

The absence of social benefits can be explained by low levels of gross domestic product per capita. Because social benefits are private benefits, cost is proportionate to the number receiving education, health care and pensions. Because social benefits are recurrent expenditure, such programmes cannot be financed by a one-off grant from the World Bank, as can capital investment in a dam or highway. When GDP per capita is a tenth or a twentieth of that of an advanced industrial society, the state lacks the tax revenue to finance such benefits.

However, the absence of civil and political rights can *not* be explained simply by reference to low levels of living standards. A number of newly industrialising countries have higher per capita incomes today than England or America did a century ago, and relatively high levels of literacy. Even more striking is the fact that a few Third World countries have established civil and political rights even though their material living standards are low relative to OECD countries or former communist regimes, or by absolute standards. India is the most notable example (Weiner and Ozbudun, 1987).

The conjunction of civil, political and social rights in one society is contingent, and cannot be taken for granted. It is perfectly possible for a society to enjoy democracy without a welfare state, or to lack democracy, or to lack all three sets of rights. As Castles (1986: 224) concludes his study of Western and communist welfare systems: 'Political choice in liberal democratic states permits of the adoption of diverse policies in response to popular demands in a way which is not possible in the communist states.'

THE INHERITANCE FROM A NON-MARKET ECONOMY

The inheritance from the past must be the starting point for thinking about welfare in an East European country today, for the collapse of a non-market economy is an ongoing process. It involves the running down of old institutions, political, economic and social, as a precondition for their replacement by new institutions.

Post-communist countries are today undergoing a fundamental transformation. In a negative sense, the revolution has already succeeded in voiding the old political order. Communist-dominated regimes have everywhere fallen, and individuals now have a significant modicum of civil and political rights. The apparatus of a repressive police state has been replaced by institutions permitting freedom of expression. Communist ruling parties have been discredited almost everywhere, including the Soviet Union. Whatever the future holds, political freedom is today widespread in Eastern Europe. Moreover, every former dictatorship has held free elections.

Much more slowly, institutions of a non-market economy are in the process of being dismantled throughout Eastern Europe. Whereas new political parties, or even a parliament, can be created overnight, it is much more difficult to create a price system where there has been none, or to create profit-making enterprises that will absorb the labour shed by the contraction of state enterprises, or to privatise enterprises that have indeterminate ownership and no accounts showing their annual profit and loss, and no balance sheet of assets and liabilities (see IMF *et al.*, 1991). The inheritance of the welfare state is also full of infirmities.

Flaws in the theory and practice of social welfare in a socialist society

Socialist societies had both material and ideal pretensions. It was claimed that a centrally planned non-market economy was materially superior to a market system in rapidly industrialising peasant societies. The absence of democracy was sometimes claimed as an economic advantage, facilitating the mobilisation of scarce resources for long-term capital investment.

Communist regimes did succeed in effectively repressing the market, thus creating enormous problems in evaluating the course of development of command economies. Planning statistics tended to concentrate upon physical quantities (e.g. tons of locomotives produced) rather than upon money values. No attention was paid to the quality of output. Services were to a large extent ignored, a matter of particular concern for social welfare (OECD, 1991). Distortions in nominal costs or prices were greater still. Charges for food and housing were set well below production costs, while monopoly prices were extracted for cars and activities free in societies with civil rights, e.g. foreign travel. Today, scholars evaluating the material state of post-communist societies do not ask how large is its national product, but how small it is (see e.g. Aslund, 1990).

Although the rulers of planned economies guaranteed everyone a job, they did not guarantee each worker enough income to support a family. In a market economy, a wage is meant to meet subsistence needs; it is the exceptional worker who is classified as in poverty. The middle mass earn enough to buy a car, buy a house, and have holidays. The overwhelming majority of persons in receipt of income-maintenance grants are unemployed or retired.

In non-market economies, the official job does not provide enough to meet a family's basic needs, let alone a Western-style living standard. Nationwide sample surveys in Czechoslovakia and Bulgaria in 1991 found that 76 per cent of Bulgarians and 56 per cent in Czechoslovakia said that earnings from their regular job are inadequate to meet their needs. The inadequacy of income was not caused by transition from a centrally planned

Table 11.2 Participation in six economies

	CFSR %	Bulgaria %
OFFICIAL *economy: legal, monetised*		
1. Official Economy or pensioner	96	90
SOCIAL *economies: non-monetised, legal*		
2. Household production	67	73
3. Help friends and relatives	76	53
UNCIVIL *economies: illegal, monetised*		
4. One or more in household in Second Economy	36	15
5. Paying connections	57	38
6. Foreign currency	29	16

Source: Nationwide Czechoslovakian and Bulgarian surveys, as reported in Rose (1991a: Table II.2).

economy but reflected continuity with conditions before 1989 (Rose, 1991a: Figure II.1; Dallago, 1990).

To attain a more or less satisfactory level of consumption, households in Eastern Europe have had to rely upon a portfolio of up to six economies, some legal, others alegal, and a third group illegal. As the Bulgarian proverb puts it, 'If you have to live from one job, you will die.' Participation in a multiplicity of economies is not unfamiliar in Western market societies, but it does not have the same meaning or scale. In Western societies, activities in the shadow economy are usually undertaken not because of economic necessity but to supplement the market economy (see Gershuny, 1979; Stark, 1989). In non-market systems, individuals may value positive aspects of do-it-yourself economic activities (growing food or home repairs), but necessity is often the spur, and people must also accept undesirable features (payment of bribes, the insecurity of alegal or illegal behaviour).

Analytically, we can define Total Economic Activity in the household as the sum of actions in six different economies (Table 11.2). The starting point is the *official economy*; it is both legal and monetised. People are paid a money wage, and their employment and earnings are officially monitored. This is the activity that accounts for official statistics about the economy; it is also the most widespread form of economic activity. However, since activities in the official economy are bureaucratically determined, it is outside the market.

Originally, the word economy referred to a *social economy*, the management of household resources without money. In Eastern Europe the root idea remains relevant. The household economy involves cooperation between members of a group bound together by ties of blood and affection;

the exchanges are literally and symbolically priceless. It is difficult for a one-person household to do all the things that can be done by a couple, or a larger family. More than two-thirds of families in Czechoslovakia and in Bulgaria rely to some extent upon household production.

The line between the household and *social exchange among friends and relatives* is an analytic distinction based on degrees of interaction and group solidarity. The deprivations and distortions of a centrally planned economy have strengthened social exchange outside the immediate household as a means of securing goods and services for about half of all households. The obligation to help other people – and the right to make claims on others – has created an extensive network of exchanges far beyond the nuclear family. Another proverb in Eastern Europe is: 'Without friends, you cannot survive.'

Social economies are not monetised. Blood relationship and friendship are the basis of claims and exchanges (see Sen, 1977; Etzioni, 1988). Insofar as there is an element of calculation, it is the expectation of receiving in return help from those whom one is helping, or from others in the same extended social network. The social economies are alegal, for they are not officially registered. Being alegal, they are not recorded. However, since no money changes hands and household work and helping others is not forbidden by law, social economies cannot be classified as illegal. From a statist perspective common to many Western as well as Eastern theories of the welfare state, such reliance expresses no confidence in the state.

Three economies are *uncivil*, for they involve cash payments that violate the law or reject state institutions. In the *second economy* people work for cash and are paid without any official record being kept. In a centrally planned system such activities are private, that is, outside the state's plan and control, and thus unofficial. But the work is in the market, involving a willing exchange of money for goods and services; it is thus a productive economic exchange. A third of all households in Czechoslovakia and a sixth in Bulgaria are in this economy. The lower Bulgarian level reflects a shortage of money, not of labour.

Paying connections is both anti-social and illegal. When power is the basis of allocation, the terms of exchange are by definition unequal. Those who have power, such as a position in the nomenklatura, can allocate desirable goods and services to themselves or use their authority to decide what other people obtain – and demand payment in return. By exploiting their authority, they are exploiting their fellow citizens in ways that are anti-social, demanding a side-payment as a condition of doing what they ought to do without it. This type of bribery and corruption is endemic in communist systems (see e.g. Kaminski, 1989; Clark and Wildavsky, 1990). More than half of all households in Czechoslovakia and nearly two-fifths in Bulgaria make some use of connections to get things done.

Dealing in foreign currencies is anti-social in a more subtle way: it denies that one's national currency has value. Since the fall of communist authorities, governments in Eastern Europe have differed in allowing the use of foreign currencies for domestic transactions, and national currencies have been volatile. When the purchase of a desirable flat or payment of a bribe must be made in a foreign currency, this is a profound vote of no confidence in the national economy, an anti-social *sauve qui peut* response to economic malfunctioning. Almost a third of households in Czechoslovakia and a fifth in Bulgaria have bought goods and services in their own country by using a foreign currency.

In non-market economies families get by through the accumulation of a portfolio of economies; 66 per cent in Czechoslovakia and 57 per cent in Bulgaria are in three or more economies. The great majority rely upon unofficial economies outside the state's control, as well as upon what the state provides. The majority say that they can get by on what they secure from a multiplicity of economies, legal and non-legal, monetised and non-monetised. But the majority are also dissatisfied with their standard of living. The modal household is both coping and dissatisfied (Rose, 1991a: 31ff, 52).

Implications for tax revenue

A centrally planned economy could appear to spend large sums on social programmes because it had a soft budget constraint (Kornai, 1980). It could manipulate prices, wages and tax revenues in order to finance programmes to its political advantage. Even if the cumulative inefficiencies were debilitating for the economy, a non-market regime did not have to worry about losing an election, for it was a one-party state.

Today, post-communist regimes face hard budget constraints if they are to meet their multiple financial obligations, such as interest payments on foreign debt, investment in infrastructure, and social welfare benefits. To fund welfare through the state, East European governments need three things: a growing economy, effective tax administration and popular support, both political and behavioural.

The state cannot fund education, health care and social security if it cannot extract the tax revenue necessary to finance these services. 'Tax administration is tax policy' (Casanegra, 1986: 18; Goode, 1984: ch. 4). Whereas the proportion of economic activity in the informal or shadow economy is of the order of 5 per cent in Western nations (see Feige, 1989), in Eastern Europe economic activity outside the tax base is much higher, for the pathologies of the centrally planned economy have made it depend upon parallel economies and vice versa (see e.g. Gabor, 1989; Grossman, 1977).

An East European optimist hopes that more than half of all economic activity is outside the fiscal purview of the state, and a pessimist fears that it is not (see Table 11.2).

Logically, a centrally planned economy can be modified only by the *contraction of government*. This could follow from the development of a civil economy independent of the state, filling the vacuum created by the collapse of a centrally planned economy. It could also happen as a consequence of the alegal second economy becoming integrated in the official economy and becoming accepted as the legal market sector of a mixed economy. This would incidentally provide a buoyant tax base to finance increased expenditure on social welfare benefits.

Where there is a tradition of a hard, oppressive state, there is a tension or conflict between encouraging the priority of fiscal advisers, increasing the tax base, and encouraging the growth of a civil economy in societies (see Tanzi, 1991). Individuals and small enterprises may justify avoidance of the official economy as a step toward freedom from abject dependence upon the official economy and allocation by the party or corrupt public officials. Behaviour that would appear uncivil in a political system in which the government respects civil and political rights might appear consistent with liberal values in a system where this tradition has been lacking.

Implications for state welfare

Throughout Eastern Europe today the heritage of corruption under communist regimes justifies distrust of the state provision of welfare. Corruption was widespread in such fields as education, health care and housing. Those in charge of delivering services could determine who got what, when and how. While no charges were levied by the state itself, public officials could and did demand money (including hard currencies) or an exchange of favours in return for admitting children to a good school, medical treatment or housing. Ideological tests could also be used for employment, for example in universities.

The governing party had no electoral incentive to curb gross abuses. Under communism, power was capital, and a position in the nomenklatura was a form of capital that could be used to produce economic benefits. Party members used their offices to secure preferential treatment for themselves, their families and their relatives in schools, hospitals and ownership of houses and flats.

Given party connivance in favouritism, absolute shortages resulting from poor economic performance and the interdependence of the illegal second economy with authority in the first economy, individuals and families had no alternative but to 'work the system' too. However, this did not leave

Table 11.3 Use of connections for welfare and consumer services

	Czechoslovakia *(% using connections)*	*Bulgaria* *(% using connections)*
Social welfare services		
Doctor	36	8
Medicine	35	12
Housing repairs	26	6
Child's education	14	2
Marketed goods		
Consumer durables	39	14
Car repairs	18	7
Other	26	2
Total using connections	64	34

Source: Nationwide sample surveys, as reported in Rose (1991b).

behind a positive picture of welfare from the state (Clark and Wildavsky, 1990). As Adam (1991: 11) has described the system in Czechoslovakia, low-paid and demoralised doctors demanded side-payments to deliver anything but perfunctory care. When tipping was seen by patients to produce better treatment, then the practice spread among better-off patients. The consequence was: 'health care ceased to be a free service to a degree; since different patients have different incomes and a different inclination towards tipping, access to health services was not equal.'

In Eastern Europe, the use of connections is widespread to obtain state welfare services as well as scarce consumer goods and services (Table 11.3). It is particularly striking that medical care, a litmus test of the welfare state in Britain, is particularly subject to the use of connections. Education is less prominent than health care because decisions about getting a youth into a selective school or university are taken less frequently and many families have no school-age children. Connections are often needed to buy such consumer durables as a television set or a refrigerator, for the scarcity of these goods enables those who control the supply to demand side-payments.

Connections are of limited importance when people can substitute their own labour or turn to the second economy, where there is a free and fair market price. In Eastern Europe people develop skills in repairing their own car and making household repairs, or else turn to friends or odd-jobs people who work for cash only. But education for one's children requires a state school and an operation requires a hospital; therefore, people who want these welfare services are more vulnerable to demands for payment.

Overall, 64 per cent of housheolds in Czechoslovakia sometimes use connections, and 44 per cent of households make a payment for using connections. In Bulgaria, the total reporting the use of connections is lower, 34 per cent; nearly everyone in this group indicates that they pay something to use a connection.

On current evidence, East Europeans fail to meet both the non-pecuniary and the fiscal conditions for the immediate and successful institutionalisation of welfare through the state along social democratic lines. Even if high tax rates were levied, the need to create a civil economy independent of the state would make it difficult to collect the revenue nominally due. In addition, there is a low expectation of government's effectiveness and low trust in the professionals who deliver services and demand side-payments. If people are to pay for welfare services, then the logic of the situation may be to reduce state subsidies to those who extract side-payments and a market that offers choice.

FREEDOM OR WELFARE FIRST?

The revolutions of 1989 sought to create a civil society, in which people have the right to think and act independently of the state, and a civil economy, in which economic activity can be independent of state control. Failure to achieve a civil society and civil economy would doom the development of a welfare state with West European standards, for there would not be sufficient revenue to finance state welfare or the honesty required to allocate it equitably.

Whereas Marshall's account of the evolution of rights appeared as uncontroversial as Clement Attlee's demeanour, the situation confronting East Europeans today is full of hard choices. People who have been deprived of freedom and of welfare now want both. While other countries in Europe demonstrate that it is possible to have both, it is not possible to achieve both at once.

Freedom as the first priority

There was a profound ambiguity in Marshall's story. It left unclear whether civil and political rights are primary values because they came first in point of time, or whether the sequence is developmental, with social rights primary because they are most recent. Elsewhere, I have argued that political and civil rights are not only primary in point of time but also first in importance (Rose, 1989: ch. 10).

Political and civil rights can be achieved extremely quickly; the deprivation of freedom in East Europe has created in reaction a demand for self-expression. In a matter of months most East European countries successfully overthrew an authoritarian regime and introduced freedom of speech, assembly and organisation and free elections. Some elected governments have gone further, showing a greater will than President Bush to risk short-term unpopularity by taking economic decisions deemed necessary though unpopular.

The rapid turn to democracy in Eastern Europe is not unique; countries of Southern Europe have earlier shown that freedom and democracy can rapidly replace dictatorship. Within a decade of the death of General Franco, a new Spanish regime successfully held three parliamentary elections, survived an attempted military coup and, the final proof of legitimacy, a government left office when it lost a general election. Portugal, Italy and Greece have each made the change from dictatorship to democracy without first achieving Northern European standards of per capita GDP or welfare. Greece provides an instructive example of a Mediterranean nation that moved from a pluralistic political system to military rule, and, when that was found inadequate and objectionable, returned to democracy.

Slow institutionalisation of a civil economy

Whereas the collapse of a totalitarian regime immediately transforms the political system, the collapse of a centrally planned economy does not instantly create a civil economy. This is a lengthy process requiring the creation of new institutions and behavioural processes at both the macro and the micro level.

In a post-centrally planned economy, the immediate issue is not the appropriate relationship between public and private sectors, but whether there is to be a private sector at all. The totalitarian system was ideologically precluded from recognising the Weberian distinction between state and non-state institutions. Multiple economies existed – but they did so without legal recognition. The first obstacle to privatisation is a recognition of the concept of a private (that is, legal non-state) sector. The Shatalin plan, rejected by President Gorbachev in 1990, recognised this. The first step called for the incorporation of state-owned enterprises as entities separate from government. Secondly, enterprises were to obtain funds on market terms, not as a first lien on the public purse. Thirdly, the enterprises were to be subject to the laws of bankruptcy, if they failed to finance themselves through the sale of goods and services (*Options*, 1990: 6).

For individuals, the first step is to survive through involvement in a portfolio of economies. Social economies, such as growing food or relying upon help from friends and relatives, do not involve money. So even if survival is achieved in an economy in transition, it is insufficient for economic growth. Many households are also active in money economies independent of the state, but, because these are alegal or even anti-social, they are not civil economies. This requires the recognition – by individuals as well as by laws and public institutions – that private economic activity is an integral part of a nation's economy. Only when the official economy incorporates the great bulk of monetised economic activity, private as well as state-owned, does there exist a civil economy.

Separate and successive steps

Given recent history, East Europeans prefer the imperfections of the present political system to a communist regime. Even if the way ahead is uncertain and a trial-and-error search involves many errors, there is no turning back to the old regime (Rose, 1991b; 1992).

In the short run, East European societies cannot achieve West European levels of welfare. Whatever they do, their living standards will remain well below that of the average OECD nation for a decade or more. To say this does not mean that they will be poor in an absolute sense, for every East European country can expect a living standard higher than that of the median member of the United Nations. Most East European nations already have a higher living standard than many OECD nations enjoyed in the 1950s or 1960s.

The growth of welfare outside the state should not be interpreted as a once-for-all unilinear shift. Just as Marshall failed to foresee Thatcher and Reagan, so we should not mistakenly project present trends in Eastern Europe forward four decades. At this point in time, the important scientific question to ask is: under what conditions could East Europeans develop a West European (that is, social democratic or social market) system?

Economic growth is a necessary but not sufficient condition for financing a welfare state; a buoyant economy must also have tax handles that effectively increase the state's revenue. Entrepreneurs who want to obtain credit or legal benefits have incentives to become integrated in the official economy. Second economy workers may want a full- or part-time job in the official economy to obtain social benefits. France and Italy demonstrate that, even in societies with a popular tradition of tax avoidance and evasion, it is possible to use organisational tax handles to collect large amounts of revenue from legally attachable employers and trading enterprises (see Rose and Karran, 1987: 54ff).

An extension of social solidarity to match the boundaries of citizenship is a second condition for extending state provision of welfare. The solidarity fostered by a totalitarian regime is that of the 'little platoon', insulating private relations from political penetration. While the social network has wide ramifications, it is based upon personal ties, not the impersonal abstraction of the state as a collective, bureaucratic provider of benefits. Even in an ethnically homogeneous East European society, the chief centralising agent, the state, represents a fearful past.

Thirdly, the state's involvement in society depends upon citizens trusting it to be honest and benign rather than corrupt and oppressive in handling funds, and delivering services. Individuals who have experienced ineffective services will have no wish to pay taxes to finance more of the same, if there is an alternative of using earnings to purchase benefits in the market. The state systems of Eastern Europe, including the welfare services, have a massive task of reorientation that could take decades to achieve.

The primary collective goal in Eastern Europe today is political, institutionalising civil and political rights where they have been absent in the past. Not only is freedom a supreme political priority, but a free system of government is more likely to be trusted to provide welfare benefits than is a regime that denies political and civil rights.

ACKNOWLEDGEMENTS

This paper is an early reflection of research on changes in Eastern Europe from a centrally politicised economy to a market economy. Surveys were supported by research grants from the National Science Foundation, Washington DC, and the Foreign Office Krowther fund. The analysis is part of an ESRC sponsored project about Social Welfare and Individual Enterprise in Post-communist Societies. The views expressed are solely those of the author.

NOTE

1 The term Eastern Europe is here a shorthand phrase to refer to the societies of Eastern and Central Europe that had centrally planned economies and were governed by an authoritarian communist regime. Today, they can be referred to collectively as post-communist systems. A reference to non-market systems emphasises one aspect of these societies; a reference to communist domination, another aspect.

REFERENCES

Adam, Jan (1991) 'Social Contract' in J. Adam (ed.) *Economic Reforms and Welfare Systems in the USSR, Poland and Hungary*, Basingstoke: Macmillan, 1–25.
Aslund, Anders (1990) 'How small is the Soviet economy?' in Henry S. Rowen and Charles Wolf Jr, *The Impoverished Superpower*, San Francisco: ICS Press, 13–61.
Baldwin, Peter (1990) *The Politics of Social Solidarity: Class Bases of the European Welfare State, 1875–1975*, Cambridge: Cambridge University Press.
Bendix, Reinhard and Rokkan, Stein (1964) 'The extension of national citizenship

to the lower classes' in R. Bendix, *Nation-building and Citizenship*, New York: John Wiley, 74–100.

Berlin, Isaiah (1969) 'On Liberty' in *Four Essays on Liberty*, Oxford: Oxford University Press.

Casanegra de Jantscher, Milka (1986) *Problems of Administering a Value-Added Tax in Developing Countries*, Washington DC: International Monetary Fund, Working Paper 86/15.

Castles, Francis G. (1986) 'Whatever happened to the communist welfare state?', *Studies in Comparative Communism* 19(3/4), 213–26.

Clark, John and Wildavsky, Aaron (1990) *The Moral Collapse of Communism: Poland as a Cautionary Tale*, San Francisco: ICS Press.

Dallago, Bruno (1990) *The Irregular Economy: the Underground Economy and the Black Labour Market*, Aldershot: Dartmouth.

Day, Patricia and Klein, Rudolf (1987) *Accountabilities: Five Public Services*, London: Tavistock.

Etzioni, Amitai (1988) *The Moral Dimension: Toward a New Economics*, New York: Free Press.

Feige, Edgar L. (1989) *The Underground Economies*, Cambridge: Cambridge University Press.

Flora, Peter J. and Heidenheimer, Arnold J. (eds) (1981) *The Development of Welfare States in Europe and America,* New Brunswick, NJ: Transaction.

Gabor, Istvan R. (1989) 'Second economy and socialism: the Hungarian experience' in E.L. Feige, *The Underground Economies*, Cambridge: Cambridge University Press, 339–60.

Gershuny, J.I. (1979) 'The informal economy: its role in post-industrial society', *Futures*, February, 3–15.

Goode, Richard (1984) *Government Finance in Developing Countries*, Washington DC: Brookings Institution.

Grossman, Gregory (1977) 'The second economy of the USSR', *Problems of Communism* 26 (5) 25–40.

Heclo, Hugh (1974) *Modern Social Politics in Britain and Sweden*, New Haven, Conn.: Yale University Press.

IMF (International Monetary Fund), World Bank, OECD, and European Bank for Reconstruction and Development, (1991) *A Study of the Soviet Economy,* Paris: OECD, vol. 1.

Institute for Public Policy Research (1991) *The Constitution of the United Kingdom*, London: IPPR.

Jimenez, Emmanuel (1987) *Pricing Policy in the Social Sectors: Cost Recovery for Education and Health in Developing Countries*, Baltimore, MD.: Johns Hopkins University Press.

Kaminski, Antoni Z. (1989) 'Coercion, corruption and reform: state and society in the Soviet-type socialist regime', *Journal of Theoretical Politics* 1 (1), 77–102.

Kornai, Janos (1980) *Economics of Shortage*, Amsterdam: North-Holland.

——— (1990) *Vision and Reality, Market and State*, Brighton: Harvester/Wheatsheaf.

Lipset, S.M. (1965) 'Introduction' in T.H. Marshall, *Class, Citizenship and Social Development*, New York: Anchor Books, v-xxii.

Lipsky, Michael (1980) *Street-Level Bureaucracy: Dilemmas of the Individual in Public Services*, New York: Russell Sage.

Marshall, T.H. (1950) *Citizenship and Social Class*, Cambridge: Cambridge University Press.

OECD (1985) *Measuring Health Care, 1960–1983: Expenditure, Costs and Performance*, Paris: OECD, Social Policy Studies No. 2.

—— (1991) *Statistics for a Market Economy*, Paris: OECD.

Options (1990) 'Steps on the road to economic reform', December, 4–8. Bulletin of the International Institute for Applied Systems Analysis, Laxenburg: Austria.

Pryor, Frederick L. (1968) *Public Expenditures in Communist and Capitalist Nations*, London: Allen & Unwin.

Rose, Richard (1976a) 'On the priorities of citizenship in the Deep South and Northern Ireland', *Journal of Politics* 38, (2) 247–91.

—— (1976b) 'On the priorities of government: a developmental analysis of public policies', *European Journal of Political Research* 4 (3), 247–89.

—— (1989) *Ordinary People in Public Policy*, London: Sage Publications.

—— (1991a) 'Is American public policy exceptional?' in Byron Shafer (ed.) *Is America Different?* New York: Oxford University Press, 187–229.

—— (1991b) *Between State and Market: Key Indicators of Transition in Eastern Europe*, Glasgow: University of Strathclyde Studies in Public Policy No) 196.

—— (1992) 'Escaping from Absolute Dissatisfaction: a Trial-and-Error Model of Change in Eastern Europe', *Journal of Theoretical Politics* 4 (4).

Rose, Richard and Garvin, Thomas, J. (1983) 'The public policy effects of independence: Ireland as a test case', *European Journal of Political Research* 11, 377–97.

Rose, Richard and Karran, T.J. (1987) *Taxation by Political Inertia*, London: Allen & Unwin.

Sen, Armartya K. (1977) 'Rational fools', *Philosophy and Public Affairs* 6 (4), 317–44.

Shlapentokh, Vladimir (1989) *Public and Private Life of the Soviet People: Changing Values in Post-Stalin Russia*, New York: Oxford University Press.

Stark, David (1989) 'Bending the bars of the iron cage: bureaucratisation and informalisation in capitalism and socialism', *Sociological Forum* 4 (4), 637–64.

Swann, Abram de (1988) *In Care of the State*, Cambridge: Polity Press.

Tanzi, Vito (1991) 'Tax reform in economies in transition: a brief introduction to the main issues', Paris: OECD conference on 'The Role of Tax Reform in Central and Eastern European Economies', 22–23 January.

Teague, Paul (1989) 'European Community labour market harmonisation', *Journal of Public Policy* 9 (1), 1–34.

Teague, Paul and Grahl, John (1991) 'The European Community Social Charter and labour market regulation', *Journal of Public Policy* 11, (2), 207–32.

Walsh, Cliff (1987) 'Individual irrationality and public policy: in search of merit/demerit policies', *Journal of Public Policy* 7 (2), 103–35.

Weiner, Myron and Ozbudun, Ergun (eds) (1987) *Competitive Elections in Developing Countries*, Durham, NC: Duke University Press.

Wilensky, Harold L. (1975) *The Welfare State and Equality*, Berkeley: University of California Press.

Name index

Subject index